Rapid Weight Loss Hypnosis

The Ultimate Guide to Lose Weight and Deep Sleep Through Meditations. Learn Hypnotherapy to Fat Burn, Fall Asleep Instantly, Increase Your Self-Esteem and Overcome Stress

By

Grace Taylor

publisher for any reparation, damages, or monetary loss due to the information herein, either directly or indirectly.

Respective authors own all copyrights not held by the publisher.

The information herein is offered for informational purposes solely, and is universal as so. The presentation of the information is without contract or any type of guarantee assurance.

The trademarks that are used are without any consent, and the publication of the trademark is without permission or backing by the trademark owner. All trademarks and brands within this book are for clarifying purposes only and are the owned by the owners themselves, not affiliated with this document.

Table of Content

PART 1

Rapid Weight Loss Hypnosis

Introduction

Losing weight and trying to maintain has always been a struggle for those wanting to do so. There are different definitions of the standard body image of males and females. Weight loss can be quick or can be achieved over time. However, losing weight faster and quicker is not healthy in the long run, but those who lose it over a period of time are more likely to retain the weight they have achieved. One of the various methods to reduce weight is hypnotherapy. This technique rewires your brain, convincing it to think that whatever method you are trying is helping you to lose weight. This type of mind-set will have a positive impact on the brain and hormonal levels, which ultimately leads to fat loss. Hypnotherapy will help you to cope up with unhealthy eating habits, control emotional eating, and keeping the cravings in control. Along with hypnotherapy, positive affirmations, meditation, enough sleep, and a positive mind-set towards your own body plays a major role in reducing weight. Hormonal levels are greatly affected by the way we think or train our minds. Recovering from a negative mind-set will help you to achieve your goal more effectively and quickly. There is also a wide range of myths that are being obeyed and followed as if they are the facts. They need to be changed or at least acknowledged to make the weight loss journey impactful and fruitful. Few of the other health benefits of hypnotherapy are dealing with the side effects of chemotherapy, cure or overcome several phobias, minimize the symptoms of inflammatory bowel disease, etc.

Chapter 01: Weight loss, Health, and Perfect Body

This chapter gives a complete insight into what weight loss is, how it works, and how it can be achieved. Also, different parameters of health and perfect body images for both genders is discussed. This chapter also focuses on the mental health as well as physical health of the person. Several factors affecting these three parameters are also discussed in detail. How a person can achieve a perfect body image is also explained how certain activities are helpful in the effort to achieve all of these with optimal results.

1.1 Weight Loss

Weight loss is a reduction of body weight owing either to deliberate (diet, exercise) conditions or to unwanted (illness). Most cases of weight loss arise from body fat loss; however, in cases of severe or extreme weight reduction, protein, as well as other substances in the body may also be depleted as well. Examples of unintended weight loss include cancer-related weight loss, malabsorption (such as from recurrent diarrheal diseases), and persistent inflammation (such as rheumatoid arthritis).

1.2 What is a healthy weight loss?

It's natural for anyone who tries to lose weight to want to lose that very fast. Although, those who slowly and consistently lose weight (about 1 to 2 pounds a week) are more effective at staying off the weight. Healthy weight loss is not just a "diet" or "program" It's about a lifelong lifestyle that involves improvements in everyday diet and workout patterns for the long term.

Once a healthy weight is achieved, make decisions based on healthy eating and exercise to allow you to keep weight off over the long term.

It's not quick to lose weight, and it requires effort. But if you're ready to get started, we have a step-by-step guide to help get you onto the road to weight loss and improved health.

Even Slight weight loss can have huge benefits

Just a moderate weight reduction of 5 to 10 percent of the overall body weight is expected to reap health benefits, such as reductions in blood pressure, blood cholesterol, and blood sugars.

If you weigh 200 pounds, for example, a weight loss of 5 percent is equivalent to 10 lbs., helping to bring your weight in check to 190 lbs. While this weight may still be within the "overweight" or "obese" range, this modest weight loss may diminish your risk factors for obesity-related chronic diseases.

So even though the end target seems to be high, see it as a trip instead of just a final destination. You will develop different ways of eating and physical exercise, which can enable you to lead a healthy lifestyle. These habits can help you keep your weight loss going through time.

Is weight reduction right for you?

Safe weight loss requires time and commitment, but you will reduce and sustain the weight for the long term by making lifestyle improvements that include a healthy diet and regular exercise.

It is a safe idea to reflect through some crucial things before making any changes:

Why do you want to lose weight? Once you've made a simple, rational, weight loss choice with a practitioner's help, it's crucial to remember that it requires time to successfully, safely decrease weight.

Do you really need to lose weight? We weren't just born to be lean or to adhere to the conception of the perfect body by culture. The size and form of your body depend on several variables, including your genetics, feeding habits, Resting Expenditure on Energy, and exercise. The main aim, when seeking to better your wellbeing, is to embrace and enjoy your body.

What is a realistic amount of weight for you to lose and maintain? Each human is special, but research indicates that losing around 1-2 pounds a week is good for success in achieving losing weight. Consult with a health care provider or certified dietitian.

1.3 Physiology of weight reduction

You have to use away more calories than you consume to reduce weight. Simple body processes (e.g., forming cells, breathing, and regulating body temperature) consume 50-70% of the calories. The Resting Energy Expenditure (REE) is the pace at which the body uses calories for specific body functions.

The REE is primarily defined by genes, gender, age, and body composition. The amount of energy consumption is set in this way. However, the sum of calories you consume each day always partially depends on how much workout you have that will impact you.

It's advised that you shed not more than 1-2 lbs. A week for healthy weight loss. You'd need to burn and/or reduce your diet by around 3500 calories, or around 500 calories a day, to lose one pound of fat each week.

How fast should you expect to lose weight?

Most exercise and diet experts believe that striving for a healthy, safe weight loss average of 1 to 11/2 lbs. A week is the best approach to lose weight. Dramatic weight loss at short notice is never safe or achievable over time. Changing food patterns, coupled with daily exercise, is the most effective means of reducing weight in the long term. It's the ideal way to make sure the weight stays off too.

Starvation or drastic diets can result in a fast weight loss, but even a rapid weight loss would be dangerous and nearly difficult for certain people to sustain. When food consumption is significantly limited (below about 1,200 calories a day), the body tends to respond to this low nutritional condition by growing its metabolic rate, eventually making weight reduction much more challenging. This often occurs as dieters indulge in meals to fast or plan to skip.

Hunger pangs, incidences of low blood sugar, aches and pains, and changes in mood from excessively strict diets can also be experienced. Binge eating and weight gain can result from these health symptoms. Because an extremely restricting diet is nearly difficult to sustain for a long period after they avoid dieting and regain their previous eating patterns, people who seek to starve themselves slim frequently continue to accumulate weight once again.

1.4 Health

Health isn't really an "absolute state of physical, emotional, and social wellness." So is not "only the lack of illness or infirmity". The first element of the term is enshrined in the popular founding document of the WHO, adopted in 1946. It was intended to have a revolutionary image of "health for everyone," one focused on an "absence" of illness that went beyond the current pessimistic definition of wellness. But in an age marked by new understandings of disease on the genetic, human, and societal rates, neither concept will do. Given that we now recognize the genome's major role in illness, even the most positive wellness promoter will certainly acknowledge the likelihood of risk-free health-being.

All said that physical, intellectual, and social interaction remains profoundly important to the present day. This framework should, in fact, be extended into two yet more dimensions. Firstly, we cannot distinguish human wellbeing from the wellbeing of our entire global diversity. In a biological vacuum, humans do not serve a purpose. In the whole of the natural planet, we live in an interdependent reality. The second dimension is within the domain of the intangible. The world of the living is dependent upon a balanced relationship with the intangible environment. Due to climate change studies, we now realize far too well how dependent our individual health-being is on the "safety" of the Earth's energy-exchange processes.

Research also added to our perception of wellbeing by an innovative procedure system that shows not just the underlying mechanisms of health problems but also signs of change. Yet science terminology may be toxic. For one, the notion of misery is no longer in vogue. It's not a technical word; it sounds abstract and old-fashioned, indicative of a period of medical impotence where people had to undergo suffering without relief or respite to accept it. Science seeks to provide the basis for removing all of what had previously happened to human misery.

Dimensions of distress are tangible, and sometimes extreme, particularly at the community level. Science has not eradicated misery, given its tremendous capacity to offer health-enhancing technologies. Becoming more positive regarding others' knowledge, rather than merely writing up reductive index cards on the state of health, unlocks the opportunity for a more rational view about what it entails to be well. The truth that in an unstable world, you can't be safe.

Health will, of course, include all diverse disease determinants. Yet to suggest this will cause a feeling of tiredness, even loss. The challenges to a minimal amount of wellbeing appear so vast and so nuanced that it is almost difficult for a single person to control their results. Yet if we have a more realistic vision of what wellbeing entails, we may be able to overcome the complexity of the illness and give clinical medicine a more concrete goal.

A French specialist, Georges Canguilhem, laid out the task most explicitly in his 1943 work, The Normal and the Pathological. Canguilhem rejected the idea of usual or unusual health problems. He saw wellness, not as a mechanistically or statistically determined item. He instead saw wellness as the flexibility to cope with one's own surroundings.

Health is not a stationary feature. It depends on their instances and differs for every person. Health is determined by the individual according to his / her practical needs, not through the physician. The doctor's objective is to assist individuals in responding to their particular current circumstances. The definition of "personalized medication" would be

The uniqueness of the health-of-normality concept of Canguilhem is that it encompasses the animate and inanimate world as well as the physical, emotional, and social aspects of human existence. It positions the actual patient in a place of self-determining control, not the doctor, to determine his or her health needs. In meeting certain requirements, the doctor is a collaborator.

Canguilhem's description is empowering for a science publication, too. A publication will change by using adaptability as the safety check to tackle the increasing conditions of the disease. The ability to adapt frees us to be flexible in the face of shifting influences that form human and community welfare. The concept of Canguilhem, therefore, helps one to adapt internationally to the disease, taking into consideration the nature of situations in a specific area, and also duration.

Health is both an inspiring idea and an elusive one. By combining excellence with adaptation, we start moving closer to a more caring, soothing, and innovative medication program — one that we will all relate to.

1.5 Types of Health

Overall, health, including physical and mental, are probably the two health types that are most frequently discussed.

Physical wellbeing frequently leads to social, mental, and financial health. Both have been related by scientific researchers to reduced stress rates and better mental and physical health.

For example, individuals with greater financial wellbeing may be less worried about finances and have the resources to more frequently purchase fresh food while those with good spiritual health can feel a sense of calmness and purpose, which power good mental health.

Physical health

Any individual with good physical health is likely to have maximum body functions and processes.

That is not only attributable to a scarcity of illnesses. Regular activity, dietary intake, and adequate rest all lead to healthier wellness. People are provided medical attention, if appropriate, to preserve the equilibrium.

Physical fitness requires following a balanced lifestyle to reduce illness incidence. For starters, sustaining physical exercise will preserve and improve a person's capacity for breathing and heart rate, muscle power, resilience, and body structure.

Pursuing good fitness and wellbeing often involves reducing the likelihood of injuries or health complications, such as:

• Minimization of occupational risks

• Using birth control when having sex

• Practice proper sanitation

• Don't use cigarettes, drink or illicit substances

• Taking the vaccines recommended for a particular disease or country when going to travel

Good physical health can function in conjunction with mental health to improve the overall quality of life for an individual.

According to a 2008 report, mental condition, for example, depression, can raise the likelihood of substance use disorders.

This will appear to have negative physical health consequences.

Mental health

As per the U.S. Health & Human Services Department, mental wellbeing relates to the physical, social, and mental wellbeing of a person. Mental wellbeing is as critical an aspect of a true, healthy lifestyle as physical health.

Defining mental wellbeing is more complicated than physical health, as certain psychiatric conditions rely on the understanding of an individual's experience.

However, with advancements in the screening, physicians can also recognize the clinical indicators of some cases of psychiatric disease in CT scans and genetic studies.

Not only is healthy emotional wellbeing characterized by the lack of stress, anxiety, or any condition. It also hinges on the ability of a person to:

• Making the most of life

• Come back from rough situations and adjust to hardship

• Balancing different aspects of life, like relationships and finances

• Stay secure and safe

• Realize one's full potential

Physical and emotional wellbeing are closely intertwined. For example, if a persistent condition impacts the capacity of a person to perform his or her daily activities, it may contribute to depression and stress. Such feelings may be related to financial or mobility issues.

A psychiatric disorder may influence body weight and physical health, such as depression or eating disorders.

An approach to "health" as a whole is important, rather than as a set of separate factors. Both forms of health are related, and as the keys to better health, citizens will strive for optimal vitality and stability.

1.6 Factors for Maintaining Good Health

Rest for Enhanced Wellness

In today's time and age, when we're short of time, rest sometimes takes the backseat to other needs, but those z's you're sacrificing right now that trigger your long-term future problems.

"Inadequate sleep has also been linked with these (obesity, diabetes, heart disease) and other health issues and is deemed as a significant factor for risk. While scientists have just begun to establish the links between inadequate sleep and disease, most experts have agreed that having enough high-quality sleep may be as critical to health and wellbeing as diet and exercise.

Some people try to get enough sleep but are prevented by an actual sleep disturbance. There are two primary categories of sleep disorders: obstructive apnea of sleep, and central apnea of sleep.

The obstructive form is the most prevalent type of sleep disorder. In obstructive sleep apnea at different possible locations, the upper airway leading to the lungs gets obstructed. This obstruction can be caused by excess tissue in the airway, such as obesity, expanded tonsils, a very large tongue, nasal congestion, and relaxation of the airway musculature while asleep.

If you are suspected of developing a sleep problem, simply contact specialists to help determine whether you are doing so and seek appropriate medication.

Sleep

Scientists have consistently advised us that most people require 7-8 hours of sleep to work effectively. But a lot of us get less than 6 hours of sleep a night now. Even lying in bed, we keep looking at our phones, or simply cannot fall asleep because we've had a very stressful day. Or nowadays, this is a huge issue, because sleep deprivation basically affects every human cell and organ system in the body. Not getting sufficient sleep is associated with obesity to diabetes, to Alzheimer's autoimmune disease. Many that usually sleep 7-8 hours at night often slow down the cycle of aging.

The keys to optimizing your sleep make it a priority that your night-time access to artificial light, maintaining a sleep-friendly atmosphere, and preparing regular meals that encourage sleep. It could be a little bowl of oats, or a buttered sweet potato, or a slice of turkey. All those things will make it easier to fall asleep.

Having fun, happiness, and purpose in life.

Lastly, maintaining a good lifestyle is genuinely essential to happiness. You may have a perfect diet, outstanding sleep, and daily workout, so what's the point if you're not happy? When you wake up every morning, you should smile and have a wonderful day ahead of you. When you're satisfied, you'll be helped by all facets of your lifestyle, and everything will come into focus.

Happiness also leads to better immune and digestive function, better sleep, and better appetite and also prevents depression. It is really necessary that you just appreciate your life every day, that you do what you do, that you are surrounded by people you want, and that you find your meaning in life. Nothing is worse than your boring day-to-day mechanical success without receiving some gratification from what you are doing. Never be afraid to pause, keep an eye on the situation, and rebuild your life/job/relationship whatever it takes. So sometimes it takes you to step out of your comfort zone, but don't be scared, it's often easier to explore to see where it leads you than never to explore

Stress management

Chronic stress affects our health profoundly, but many of us simply ignore it. This is terrible, since no matter what lifestyle you adopt, how frequently you work out, and what vitamins you take if you don't control the stress, you'll always be at risk for chronic degenerative disorders such as cardiac failure, diabetes, thyroid issues, and an autoimmune disorder.

Seek to maintain good mental wellbeing and harmful thinking and feelings will potentially affect your body function and harm the body in a certain way.

You will have your ups and downs, but it's much better overall to have a positive attitude about your life. Also, keep an eye on your spine's health, which is easiest to do by stretching yoga every day. Chiropractors often test the spine for good balance and stability due to the nervous system impacts it has. Via the nervous system, the brain interacts with the body. Health issues may emerge if there is an issue with this link.

Often, you should try meditation and learn to be conscious. It's not for everybody, but everybody can try it. You never realize you can really enjoy it and change your way of thinking and feeling about your experiences, especially stressful ones. Pay heed to the emotions, desires, and perceptions of the body to become consciously mindful of them, and to be able to control them properly as it helps to achieve balance in a fast-paced modern environment.

Neuroscientific findings suggest that meditation improves blood flow, decreases blood pressure, and prevents individuals at risk of developing hypertension: it often lowers coronary disease incidence and frequency, and the likelihood of dying from it.

People become less prone to get trapped in stress and fatigue, so they become more able to manage their behavior. We don't really know how to pay close attention to what we're doing with our busy speedy lives, and we skip entire pieces of our lives, interactions, and quickly get wrapped up in over-thinking – destroying our wellbeing and leaving us frustrated and tired.

Practice Good Posture

When talking about strategies to promote optimum fitness, posture is definitely not something that people really much worry about. We should, however! "Being bad in posture will place more stress on some muscles and joints, causing them to overwork and fatigue them. This shows that poor posture can cause tiredness, circulatory system, joint problems, emotional state, musculoskeletal impairment, jaw pain, breathing effectiveness, headaches, sexual function, and pain in the shoulder and back.

Establish Exercise Habits – Foundational for Maintaining Good Health

There are seven of these explanations why exercise is important to preserving good health:

1. Weight Control

2. Combat health problems and diseases

3. Improves mood

4. Energy improves

5. Gives decent sleep

6. Underpins a balanced sex life

7. it's fun, social and puts down stress

It's also necessary to contact a doctor before initiating an exercise routine to make sure you're safe for all levels/forms of training.

Moderate aerobic activity for not less than 150 minutes per week or 75 minutes a week of vigorous aerobic activity a week is recommended, or a combination of the two.

Do not forget to use free weights, weight machines, or body-weight workouts to integrate strength training for all the main muscle groups at least twice a week.

Spread the work out during the week.

Genetic factors

Each individual has a range of genes when born. In some people, an unexpected genetic sequence or change may lead to a healthy level that is less than optimal. People can inherit the gene from each parent, which increases their risk to certain conditions of health.

Environmental factors

Environmental factors have a major role to play in wellbeing. The environment alone sometimes suffices for health impacts. Many times, an environmental stimulus in an individual who has an elevated hereditary risk of a certain disorder will induce illness.

Access to health care plays a part, but the WHO suggests that the following factors can influence health more significantly than this:

• Where an individual lives

• The state of the environment around us

• Human genetics

• Earnings

• Their education level;

• Place of work

These may be classified as follows:

The physical environment: This involves growing germs that occur in an environment, as well as the rates of pollution.

The social and economic environment: That can involve a community and family's financial standing, as well as societal culture and relationship efficiency.

A person's characteristics and behaviors: Genetic composition and lifestyle decisions for an individual may have an effect on their general wellbeing.

Perfect Body Image

Everyone has a very different view of the ideal body image, but we are highly affected by the expectations of culture and the media. The expectations of society hues our views about the perfect body image, and this occasionally poses issues or causes suffering.

Society's Idea of the Perfect Body Image

Society suggests to us what body appearance we will be looking for. We see pictures of flawless bodies everywhere over us, on TV, in film, in magazines and newspaper advertisements and digitally. Reporters and gossip columnists also report about people's presence in the press and political figures. How much do you see posts about the hairstyle of Hillary Clinton or the outfit of Michelle Obama? They really aren't professional models, and their appearance is not important to any of their jobs, yet it is a common discussion topic. No wonder so many people are concerned about getting the right body image portrayed!

The reality is that individuals come in all shapes and sizes and can be appealing to people of all shapes and sizes. In reality, curvy women have been seen as more desirable in recent years than really slim women. That, however, is no longer true nowadays.

The Ideal Body Image for Men

The typical American male is approximately 5'9 "according to the National Center for Health Statistics, and weighing approximately 190 lbs. However, the typical male fashion model is only 6'1 "in height and just weighing only 160 lbs. It's not as shockingly slim as female models, but it's much thinner than the normal man. Male models, of course, typically work out and often have well-defined muscles. Sadly, people often see these images and believe this is the ideal body image.

The Ideal Body Image for Women

When we accept the conception of the culture focused around the stereotypical media picture about the ideal body image for women, we would assume that the perfect woman was around 5'10 "and weighed just 120 lbs. However, as per the National Center for Health Information, the typical American woman is just about 5'4 "and weighing approximately 169 lbs. There is a considerable discrepancy there. Women's model picture also advises us people should be white, tan, and have huge breasts. She should be young, and a little athletic, of course. She should have no physical impairments. If she is smart, it doesn't matter that much, as long as she's visually attractive.

Drawbacks of Tempting for the Perfect Body Image

Most of us aspire to remain safe and are well conscious of the dangers of obesity. It is essential to remember, though, that the perfect body picture portrayed by mass media isn't safe. The average fashion icon, weighing only 120 lbs, has a body mass index of 17.2, and physicians find something below 18.5 underweight. Getting overweight is dangerous, but being underweight is also harmful. Anaemia, nutritional deficiency, osteoporosis, cardiac attacks, increased vulnerability to illness and infection, and slow wound healing is dangers correlated with being underweight.

In an effort to suit the advertisements they see, people who wrongly think media photographs reflect a healthy weight or good health may diet unnecessarily. Eating problems such as anorexia or bulimia also occur in certain individuals. Obviously, individuals with anorexia and bulimia are not healthy, and most people will accept that people who are extremely underweight are not really desirable, either. However, people with eating disorders often have distorted images of the body. They genuinely think they are overweight and disgusting even though they aren't.

It's possible a good woman's body will remain slender in the foreseeable future. And for this there are many reasons:

Globalization

Television and the internet became widespread worldwide. Plump women have also been respected by the conservative cultures of Puerto Rico, Samoa, and Tanzania. They started to interpret chubbiness as something hideous, however, beginning in the 1990s, having been inspired by European countries.

The images of powerful and heavy people are often respected in rural areas, where manual work often counts. However, people moving from villages to cities are starting to shift their attitudes towards more slender women.

The media industry is for skinny girls

Very commonly, fashion designers choose slim girls (sometimes with a common boyish appearance) as they look amazing in any garment. Since they deal with computer programs, they are able not only to build slender bodies but even body forms that literally cannot exist.

At the same time, statistics show that a teenage girl gets 180 minutes of information from different media every day, while she spends only 10 minutes conversing with her family members. So unrealistic beauty standards are progressively being incorporated into our consciousness and our children's awareness.

Of course, some women and plus-size models have somewhat affected fashion, but the effect is unlikely to be long-lasting. In comparison, fashion designers tend to create clothing with an "hourglass" body image while avoiding certain forms of feminine bodies. The number of inhabitants of the glamorous half of the world who have the preferred forms of fashion designers is no more than 8 percent of the nation.

Hourglass figure for women

A slim waist and wide hips are likely to stay among their preferences. Yet, due to the power of the apparel industry, the preference for thin girls would stay more fashionable.

Relative satiety of the population

As we have pointed out, people want more thin women because there is no fighting or famine. And because most developed world countries have ample food to consume, they would equate chubby shapes with obesity.

Removing borders between genders

More and more people continue to become heterosexual, including celebrities, influenced by the idea of feminism. They think there should be no difference between male and female, so they begin to wear masculine hairstyles and clothing. It is upon you to determine if it is good or bad, but the feminine appearance standard is likely to skip any gender markers in the foreseeable term.

1.7 How to love your body?

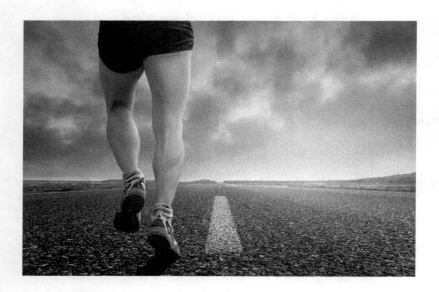

Meditation

Meditation is a nice means of centring yourself. You should still switch to meditation when life gets difficult, or if the mind gets pounding. It is open to everyone as well since you can do it everywhere. All you have to do is find a peaceful and relaxing space, shut your eyes, and just take a breath.

Slow down

We live in this fast-paced world. Let yourself calm down, appreciate the memorable times, and take care of yourself. Here are a few various perspectives to help your everyday life

slow down.

Eat slowly. Make it a priority to sit at a table at every meal you eat, without disturbances. And ensure that you carefully chew, and really enjoy what you consume. That basic exercise is a game-changer on what you experience every day inside your body.

Rest. If you can tell your body or mind is overly drained, then it is vital that you encourage yourself to give your body what it wants. Everything right is to go to bed early without doing the dishes. It is fine to miss the exercise, and you can get home early and veg out on the sofa. Letting the body rest is Fine. It's the vessel, after all, that takes us through every moment — it needs your support and affection. Relaxing in your own way can help you revive your body much quicker and feel healthy.

Breathe. Take a few minutes of the day and simply relax. Take 10 deep breathing exercises to let the body tune in. Once you go forward with your everyday activities, let yourself re-center and concentrate.

Mirror work

Every day, you gaze into the mirror. To others, that may be a very unpleasant event due to the unkind inner voice, which you witness. Don't mind these terms. Instead, once you look

in the mirror, look in the eyes, and tell, "I love you." Do this, even if you feel stupid!

Self-talk has been shown to be effective. Positive, love messages can also be put up with a few comments on your mirror. Awaking each day with a kind and supportive note to yourself and your body can shift the most positive way in which you have a connection with yourself.

Dare to not compare your body.

"If you compare yourself to other people, you will build a million excuses that you would dislike your body. Relating yourself to someone often makes you feel bad and miserable with your own body, so try not to do so. Your body might not be flawless relative to a celebrity or friend, but it's the only body you'll ever get. You would rather accept this fact and love your body the way it is than waste your time hating any part of it."

Be your body's best friend.

You must actually talk to yourself and try to treat yourself as you would be talking to your best friend. If your best friend missed a workout or gained a few pounds, you'd encourage her to get back on the right track — not start judging her. Fitting bottoms, after all, come in different shapes and sizes.

Focus on what helps you feel good.

Stop looking at taking care of your body as a chore. You have to let go of a stupid ideal goal that is harder and harder to achieve at the age of 32 without going back to a boring stereotype. Diet and exercise-related are less to the ideal of someone else and more to what is ideal for you. Eat healthy food because it makes you feel good, and stay away from anything that makes you feel guilty or unhappy or sick. Run or workout as it allows you to be more creative and productive at work and a more affectionate partner and enhances the standard of living. This type of treatment is good enough to justify whether it makes you thinner or not.

Gratitude

Getting a regular routine devoted to appreciation is a great way of enhancing your self-love. And all you need to do is begin journaling.

When waking up each morning and every night until you go to sleep, note down three items that you are thankful for. It's a beautiful way of loving yourself and living. It's a great moment to show gratitude to your body!

Mindful movement

Moving your body in a tactful way is a lot different from

exercising or working out. It's not about getting yourself forced to do something you hate. It's about keeping your body-oriented and telling yourself what you like.

Find a way to function, which can help the body and mind feel good. Maybe you're aiming for a run or a yoga class? If you haven't found your choice of mindful movement, keep searching. Because the best part you can find is that you can choose something you cherish.

Step off the scale.

Knowing how to respect the body and embrace everything brilliance and imperfections — is a progression and an expedition but one well worth it.

If body positivity isn't working for you, go for body neutrality.

When you sound inauthentic about going right into the good feelings, that's fine. First, move on towards your body's neutral thoughts.

"If your thinking is 'my stomach feels gross,' it is impossible to convince yourself that your stomach is always perfect. However, you should practice the idea: 'This is a human stomach' anytime you glance at it or if your subconscious starts to think about it. 'The longer you practice these kinds of rational thinking transfers, the better they get—the faster they ultimately become the normal, natural feelings.'

For people battling positive body image, body neutrality may be unexpectedly empowering.

Chapter 02: Role of Human Mind in weight gain/loss

This chapter discusses in detail how a human brain can deceive you for gaining or losing weight. Triggers of overeating or undereating are discussed in this chapter. In order to attain optimal health, one should have a good relationship with food. Food should always be considered as a pleasant or joyful thing rather than giving it a name like food to reduce fat etc. This chapter will help you to overcome the negativity which you have for yourself so that you can live life to its fullest.

2.1 The brain does make you fat

Excess weight may feel like a thing of the belly, but your nervous system is among the major barriers to losing. What you feed, look and respond affects you whether or not you add weight. This is how the subconscious controls the body — and what you can do about it.

Anxiety fuels your needs.

Have a big presentation already come up, or are you about to have a challenging conversation with somebody you love? You should seek to control the discomfort; otherwise, you can catch yourself stopping the dinner otherwise preferred snack for a second. Sometimes referred to as stress feeding, fear causes this form of action and, when treated, may be counterproductive to the scale — both upward and downward. Fear may have an overwhelming impact on the diet. Anxiety occurs differently in persons. Certain people will find themselves trying to regulate any ounce of food they consume, some may have the need to overeat, while some may lose their desire to eat completely.

Allowing negative to dominate

Within the head, the crystal-half-empty mentality may be challenging, but it often causes unhealthy habits of eating. Losing weight marketing is especially good at people who prey on the poor ways of thought that most people form about food. The whole food industry is built to make consumers feel terrible for their health and make them believe they ought to waste all this money for a diet program that doesn't function. Whenever the person's diet crashes, they feel bad for themselves and the process begins. People sometimes fault themselves for failing the diet, not the guy, when in fact it is. Before people get free of their eating habits, the body is hard to understand and everything that it offers, doesn't matter what big it might be.

Your brain turns dieting into fat preservation.

There are numerous misconceptions out there about weight reduction, but one aspect that is unequivocally real is that the brain avoids diet. Key brain cells actively prevent fat burning in the body when food is rare. A group of neurons in the brain coordinates appetite and energy spending and can turn on and off a switch to consuming or backup calories depending on what's in the environment available. We help us feed if food is abundant, and if food is unavailable, we transform our body into a survival mode to avoid us from losing fat.

Depression triggers eating

Thinking processes causing obesity may be unconscious, but stress is an evident road to eating disorders. The weight gain is immutably related to the anxiety condition. Anxiety can significantly shift the culinary attitude and viewpoint. Depression feelings can manifest in excessive feeding or deprivation so what's important is resolving the head-on feelings. Recognizing what is going on is so crucial, and finding professional treatment so that you really can take action not to allow stress to affect your well-being and weight.

Work destroys weight reduction targets

Life is insane, so force oneself to go to the gym to stop those a.m. while you are counting calories. You can sense the cravings much more depressed than usual. And a brain under tension will indirectly weaken your attempts. If people feel uncomfortable regarding their bodies and eating patterns, the kinds of food they consume or the volume they consume can be unnecessarily limited. The body is created to live. It doesn't realize why the human intentionally limits food, it only recognizes but it does not have sufficient, and it naturally slows down functions of the body, like metabolism, to save energy and to live. This physiological cycle often starts a primary urge to consume more to live, causing the individual to over-feed and struggle over food unconsciously.

Denying pleasure

Part of the weight-loss challenge is what products you choose to go there. If you're carelessly going for an apple because it's nice for you, however, it gives you a stomach ache, why don't you make a move to eat a mango you'd like more? Think about consuming an experience rather than a need. What that means is that by having the time to reflect on what you actually want to consume and make it a conscious activity, you allow yourself the chance to tune in and adapt to the nutritious meals that you would want to buy and enjoy, leaving you happy at mealtime.

Being judgmental

Will you feel a bad or a favorable connotation when you speak about a greasy burger and fries? How about a simple salad with hardly any treats? As we mature and start to assign various names to specific items, we start naming them accidentally — and sometimes, mindlessly —. **Eliminating a** 'good' behind such dishes and the 'evil' behind them will help shift the emphasis. "Food has little meaning, so feeding is not white and black. It has far less control over you, until food has little moral obligation.

You don't even ask why

You remind yourself of something before you place the donut in your stomach. Is it food you desire — or anything else? "Enquire oneself if meal is even whatever you need. People often crave comfort and support when eating without body hunger. It's fine to eat at a family party for selfish reasons, like cake, but you have to be capable to identify those signs and make a decision for yourself whether food is that you need or want or whether anything else will assist you

accordingly.

Just to tap into gratitude

Humility can boost your well-being in several respects, but it's difficult to be thankful to oneself. Whenever an eating spree begins a cycle of shame, look at how incredible it is our brain and heart function to keep us healthy instead of throwing themselves a hard time. It gives sense why, if we build shortages by dieting, certain biological forces be in high gear to save our resources and lead us to search for high-calorie foods — or normally foods that we've resisted. What if we all quit dieting nonsense and chose to take control of our body and function through our appetite rather than battle it? Instead, in a range of body types and ages, we will find much healthier individuals who kept fairly healthy weights and enjoyed improved fitness.

Confidence won't support you

If you really can't turn your mind the correct way around? And do not be scared to ask somebody who is able to tackle something that delays your development, for assistance. Trying to break the dietary and food anxiety mental loop is challenging, it requires training and experience. A nutritionist who specializes in mindful eating as well as the – anti-diet

method will assist you on the journey.

2.2 How to lose weight using your mind?

If you've ever attempted weight reduction, you realize that consuming nutritious food and exercising your body are essential elements of every weight-loss strategy. Yet have you learned that reaching or sustaining a balanced body structure exists both in the body and mind? In fact, if you've repeatedly tried to lose some weight but never succeeded or you lose the weight and then regain the weight (and then some!), your thoughts and beliefs — not your diet — are most likely holding you back. This is because the extra weight is a result of the state of mind or sentiment. And the main reason people struggle to lose weight is that they ignore to implement adjustments in their subconscious mind in order to support their conscious objectives.

2.3 How to Reshape Your Figure with Your Thoughts

Listen to your self-talk.

Self-respect and recognition of oneself are the key elements for reaching optimum weight. Yet, most individuals cannot lose weight when participating in body-shaming talk and actions. It's crucial to learn if you spoke about yourself before attempting to lose weight. Whether you tell your body you dislike how it appears for much of your life, or scratch your face in the mirror in frustration that someone used to do that to you, the subconscious mind would accept the emotional conditioning. You will reconfigure your subconscious mind by communicating with your body in a constructive, caring manner — the way you'd be communicating to an innocent kid. Look in the mirror to see what the body likes. Touch the parts you want to change, and say, "Thank you for keeping me alive." Make sure your body loses weight safely. Perform so every single day. Through time, the subconscious can comply with the urge to shed weight, actively.

Say affirmations.

Affirmations tend to reinforce your trust in the latest tale; you are designing the subconscious. When they are convincing, they do work well. Yet if you think, "I'm going to be 80 pounds thinner in a month," your amygdala won't accept it. Instead, try to say, "I become the super fit person that lives inside me! "And claim, 'I'm making good choices now that reflect my ideal weight.' You might also create a routine of voicing your comments.

For example, you can smudge stagnant energy in your room or home, light candles, sit with your closed eyes, and say your statements 3 times in a row. Practice this two to three times a day. You may want to repeat another variation of your comments right before you feel sleepy when your subconscious mind is more open to advise. Remember, the affirmations have to be as if they had already manifested in the present tense. Affirmations will not trigger something to happen. They accept everything.

Try Tapping.

The Emotional Freedom Technique (EFT) or Tapping, helps match the subconscious mind with the expectations on an optimistic basis by resolving the unconscious feelings, habits, values, traumas, and more than that contribute to weight gain. You begin by stating your current restricting conviction preceded by expressing how you enjoy and support yourself while taping on different points of acupressure. For starters, you might claim, "I love and truly support myself even if I have a difficult time trying to lose weight." This removes stress levels in the body and can remove the negative emotions and values connected with the extra pounds, and you can break old patterns and recover.

Identify Your 'Trouble Thoughts'

Identify the thoughts that cause you trouble and fight to eliminate and alter it. Maybe if you look into a mirror, it's your inner voice. Or cravings when stressed out. Let them avoid knowingly by telling 'no' out loud. It may sound silly, but that simple action breaks your chain of thought and allows you to introduce something new or healthier one. The best approach to do this is to count as many as you need from one to 100 times until the damaging thoughts fade.

Eat mindfully.

Research suggests that stress reduction — concentrated knowledge of your emotions, behaviors, and intentions — plays an important role in weight reduction in the long term when combined alongside certain weight loss approaches. Learn alertness when you cook and enjoy your food. Seek to be aware of starvation and plenitude thoughts. Pay close attention to flavors, textures, and the munching as well as gulping actions of your food. Be conscious also of how the body sounds after consuming those foods. This exercise will help lower binge and raise an understanding of behaviors that do not benefit the weight-loss goals. So if you try to connect what you eat to how you feel, you're not going to have to eat normally to lose weight. It is going to happen mercilessly. Also, your body composition and body image will be transformed when you learn from your mistakes about food as body-nourishment. When you link with your body and nurture it from an area of empathy and self-respect, the emotions focused on self-respect create in your body a metabolic environment conducive to ideal fat burning.

Address Yourself Like You Would a Friend

We are extremely tough on ourselves whenever it comes to beauty ideals and body image. The expectations we set for ourselves are harsh. So we should never have kept many of those requirements to our peers or loved ones. You receive the same consideration so kindness as everyone else; handle yourself like that.

Throw Out the Calendar

Patience is also important when you lose weight in a healthy and sustainable matter. Plus, if you focus on achieving genuinely actionable goals, such as taking 10,000 steps each day, and no need to get tangled up in a timeline of goals ahead.

Say "good-bye" to Energy Vampires.

One of the most striking things that have been observed in the relationships among both vampires and sensitive people is the discrepancy in their tendencies to gain weight. Your life and relationships represent your capacity to nurture oneself. If you are in a variant relationship where you constantly give and try to please some other individual, your efforts to lose weight will become in vain because you are using on the energy of your vampire (which can be a state — not a person). This causes even more stress and cortisol and takes your own energy. As a result, you look out for sugar, carbs, and/or alcohol. And you will keep on gaining weight no matter what you do — even when you eliminate the carbohydrates because the weight acts as an extra layer of "self-protection.

Take a Breath

Taking a few minutes of stability at the beginning of your workout, or even at the beginning of your day, slowing down and simply focusing on the act of breathing can help you create your intentions, link with your body, and even lower the response to the stress of your body. Lie down with legs stretched and place one hand on your stomach and one on your chest. Inhale for four seconds, hold for two and then exhale through the mouth for six seconds. With each breath, the hand kept on your stomach should be the only one to rise or fall.

Focus on the Attainable

If you have never been to a gym before, your goal shouldn't be to do 30 minutes on the elliptical on the first day. A better goal might be to go out for a 20-minute walk. If you want to cook more often but have little or no experience with healthy recipes, don't expect to find specific healthy recipes every night after work.

Weight Loss and Psychology: Why Your Brain Might be keeping you from losing weight

Designed to Eat

So why is it really so hard to reduce weight? The human body and brain are meant to eat — explaining why weight loss proves so difficult for so many people. The factors of obesity are complicated. Obesity is not merely a laziness trait or an indicator of mental dysfunction. Therefore, hereditary and biological influences do not function in isolation but work with a variety of environmental variables on a permanent basis. Both the accessibility and persuasive advertising of unsafe food contribute to the epidemic of obesity.

2.4 Why Is Changing Eating Habits So Difficult?

Although environmental and genetic influences play a part,

no-one demands whether individuals be liable for their everyday choices on when and how much to consume. And why do we catch ourselves slipping back into the old ones after making up our intention to break a habit? How can't we just make a choice and move on with it? What challenges and infuriates those seeking to lose some weight is why it is too damn hard to alter one's eating patterns.

A crucial part of the issue is that we think we have much more power over our behavior and attitude than we actually do. Stress, fear, and temptation will constrain the deliberate control of our decisions.

What drives our actions is not reasoning, but the biochemistry of the brain, habits, and addiction, consciousness states, and what we see people doing around us. We're emotional creatures with the capacity to justify — not emotionally reasonable beings. If we're anxious, miserable, or addicted, no matter how well the advice we get, there's a chance we won't be able to act on that. In general, the more ancient, emotional brain has priority over the more logical, newer brain.

But even though we excluded certain individuals that are nervous, anxious, or obese from the study sample, we will still be left with a huge number of individuals that can't hold to their commitment to losing weight.

One explanation is about different personalities. Another is that determination isn't constant. Resolve ebbs and falls, like the water. Every second we may be charged up to be mindful of our diet, but our attitude, our state of mind, or meaning has shifted in the next instance. We find ourselves wallowing in unhealthy treatments, much to our great annoyance.

We can convince ourselves to do just about anything we want to do — especially when our minds are used to doing the behaviors. But it's not easy to try to convince ourselves to do things we really don't want to do — behaviors our brain isn't used to — We are highly skilled in making fantastic (and credible) justifications about why we can't do what we don't really want.

Transformation is daunting, and anybody who discovers a way to inspire and self-discipline upon a bottle and the industry would make a lot. Nonetheless, the next greatest part is useful observations into the mechanism of improving our behavior, despite the absence of such an action.

In the end, our core emotional principles will determine our choices, for better or worse. If we recognize our true interests, we will use them to build a balanced lifestyle that represents the best of ourselves. Our deepest principles can be called upon to hold us on track, particularly when we are faced with temptations and disruptions. When we go down the wrong path, they may even act as our guide.

Whether we are willing to remain assiduously dedicated to our emotional values, we can rest assured that our health and fitness goals will be achieved. And if we do, some of us may go a step further and support friends and family members so that they can join us in being happier and healthier.

2.5 Weight Loss: How to Reset/Refresh Your Brain for Success

How a dieting behavior keeps the weight on?

We have all been here — after a week on a New Year's diet of being "healthy," you're having a celebration for the great game that is filled with sweets. Suddenly you call your name chili dip and corn chips, and you can't focus on a game as you are utilizing all your body energy avoiding chips. You experience remorse, embarrassment, and diminished self-esteem as you eventually give way.

Combine these thoughts with the fact that you may as well consume more as you've ruined your diet before you went back to being "normal" tomorrow, and you've added weight.

When we limit our food eating, several things happen in our bodies. We know our metabolism is slowing, and the cells that control our feelings of fulfilment and hunger are getting out of knock. You wind up consuming so much, not because you're poor or frail, but due to your body wants everything this can to break out of the self-imposed food shortage.

Many experiments have displayed that a restrictive diet eventually results in gain of weight, not losing it. But researches also have found that self-esteem may guess dieting results.

You continue to build healthier dietary behaviors in the long run by trying to raise the culpability and guilt around diet and a greater understanding of body identity.

Your brain is on a nutrition but not your stomach

Your dietary mind-set may even enable you to take more food or gain weight even if you're not actively on a diet plan. You that consume more than you will usually eat, expecting you'll again start a restricted diet early.

Our bodies can be much more equipped to thrive in periods of drought, from an evolutionary viewpoint. The yo-yo dieter's body is habitual to random times of restriction or food shortage; hence the body strives to store and eat more in general. The body of humans doesn't want weight reduction, and it battles back.

You're also told by a dietary mind-set that choices of your food reflect your value as a human being. You consume "evil" things, and you're a cruel guy or a poor person or an incompetent one. This can reinforce an emotional eating cycle, which reduces self-esteem, adds extra weight, and is hard to break.

Work on your negative self-talk.

If we attach our self-worth too closely to our food preferences and pair it with a rigid diet, we set ourselves up to struggle and feel bad, which in effect causes unhealthy eating habits and then more shame. Write down the positive changes you make every day in a journal (such as drinking more water or taking a walk), and stop using the words "good" and "bad" to describe your dietary choices — and oneself.

Ultimately, what works for long-term weight loss is minor, radical steps to your overall eating patterns. The less you concentrate on filtering and categorizing items, and the better you work on developing a balanced diet and fitness habits, the safer the body — and mind — can become.

2.6 How to change your mind-set toward food?

Believe in your vision.

That's just so important. There's no point in having a view unless you believe it could become a reality. For all, you have to trust that you will make this happen. That you can change your attitude, lose weight, and wait for a better life.

Another thing to remember is that when you crush goals, some individuals could become envious. Changing habits takes a lot of work because not everyone is prepared to put this sort of effort into it. And if fundamentally they want the very same thing, their attitude may be somewhat specific. That's fine. Don't become disrupted by insecurities of other people.

Hold the dream upfront and genuinely think it is searching for you. That'll help you stay focused and keep moving on.

Believe you are in control.

You have to take accountability for your decisions to excel in reducing weight, among other objectives – you have to trust that you are in charge. If you put your fate in other people's

hands, but you'll never be able to move on. Of course, there always will be circumstances beyond our power, but we choose to react – that's up to us.

Envision a better life.

So what would life be like if you put good habits in place? Will you be at home with your clothing and shoes? Will a new dress help you feel sexy? Will that offer you more energy? Can you ever feel better? More laughs? Just to feel happier? Will you make a better mother, a wife, a girlfriend, a partner, and a spouse? Seek to get as thorough and realistic as possible? What would make it easier if you changed your lifestyle?

Take time to imagine a happier future in the start, and during your weight loss. It may be challenging to alter our behaviors and why to bother if it doesn't take us to something different and better. Imagine a happier future that will give us everything to look forward to and aspire for.

Remove clutter and chaos.

It's really tough to imagine a happier future while you constantly surrounded by chaos and confusion. Chaos and clutter create hot zones, and it's difficult to ascertain new habits and routines when trying to survive hot zones. Hot

zones are instances when you're tired out, swamped, and the choices taken are more about having survived the moment rather than concentrating on long - term goals.

Be grateful.

Showing gratitude for everything that life gives us is so extremely important. All the events that annoy or harm us are lessons gained. To be appreciative helps to keep us down to earth and grateful for the hard work it takes to achieve objectives. It's saying thank you to the world for honoring efforts. In my knowledge, appreciation is a mental change that can bring you to the greatest and toughest moments in your life.

If you're struggling to make lifestyle changes or push through difficult times, simply take time every day and trying to think out 1-3're grateful for, like really incredibly thankful. Think of lessons gained and how you will get stronger because of it. Life is small, or long, so being thankful can make you enjoy what you have rather than dwelling on the unpleasant.

Focus on solutions, not excuses.

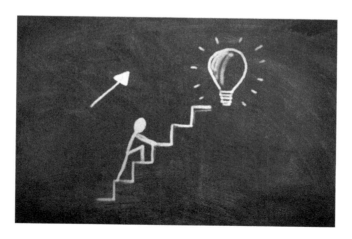

A mindful tactic that would have been very beneficial throughout one's weight loss program is trying to focus on alternatives rather than rationalizations. Excuses fulfill three functions. First, we use reasons, and we're afraid to lose. So rather than having failed at a workout regimen, we say something like, "I can't go into the gym at a certain time" or "I'm tired" or "Those workouts haven't ever worked for me. This gives us a chance to release up or not pursue it. But failing is part of the journey. It's alright to collapse. And instead of granting yourself the chance to give up, grant yourself consent to try. In order to be fortunate, not just at losing weight but also in life generally, you have to be okay with failings. Understand fall nine times get up 10.

Second, we use arguments when we are sluggish. Note, this is going to be on the harder love line. It's not that don't get lazy but don't take this as self-righteous. Yet take a good look at your justifications. Is it because you just can't do "fill in the blank" or is it just you do not feel like doing "fill in the blank.

Third, we aren't ready for a transformation. Definitely, we claim we would like to lose some weight, but our excuses speak differently. We aren't willing to change our food patterns, focus on improving workout, get hold of the hot zones, and make the time to plan and prep meals. Even though we'd like to slip it into a pair of skinny jeans, and have much more power, in reality, we're comfortable where we're

at. And instead of stepping beyond our comfort bubble, we start making excuses.

Learn to cope.

Many of our issues with weight loss derive from our physiological responses to tension. How many times you have been craving pasta or chocolate because you were having a bad day. Or ate pizza because there's nothing to prepare for the meal, and the kids start yelling. Or giving up on losing weight because the job is stressful when the children have a million things or some other exhausting season of life.

When you want to drop weight, life doesn't begin the path automatically, and pain disappears. Nope, sadly life will never be ideal, and there will always be stress. Therefore, if you slip off track each time, life does not go your way, then it is time to learn new strategies for coping. The goal is to maintain a healthy lifestyle and lose weight, given the obstacles life throws our way.

The great news is many of the techniques for weight loss also strive to help manage the stress. For instance, meal planning and meal prep help when we are busy at work and tasks to have food ready for eating during the week. Exercising makes us happier in more respects than anyone can count. You gain

more nutrients from consuming smoothies and eating fewer fried foods than any sum of coffee.

If the way you cope with stress prevents you from putting new habits in place or maintaining them, then discussion with a therapist or counselor is highly recommended. A therapist or psychologist may help you build better communication strategies and function through the pain. This will enable you to clear up space in your mind to focus on the happier existence.

Plan it, be prepared, and take action.

Sometimes we look enviously at someone who has achieved weight reduction targets (or other objectives) and conclude it was convenient for them. Quite possibly, they failed much like everyone else. They had problems and losses. The distinction being they kept it up – they kept going amid the obstacles. We can't equate someone's Day 1 to another's Day 300. There are a lot of sweat, blood, hard work, and tears that can happen in 299 days.

In order to enjoy achievement, you have to develop a plan, implement change, and then take measures. A new, better quality of life will not happen without any of those 3 things.

Chapter 03: Role of Human Body in weight gain/loss

After looking into the role of the human mind in gaining or losing weight now comes the human body itself for the same purpose. As there are several hormones that trigger hunger or suppress the hunger mainly because of how you feel about it. If you keep on stressing for weight loss, your body will release the stress hormone, which ultimately results in retaining the weight and in worst scenarios, it starts storing the energy in the form of fats. This chapter is a complete guide of how the body plays an important and vital role in regulating body weight. Emotions are the major factor that impacts the human body as well as mind.

3.1 Fix the Hormones to Control Your Weight

One's weight is controlled largely by hormone levels. Hormones affect your desire to eat, and the amount of fat you store. Here are nine ways to "fix" the hormone levels controlling your weight.

Insulin is released by the pancreatic beta-cells. It's secreted during the day in tiny quantities and during meals in greater amounts. Insulin enables your cells to take energy or storage in blood sugar, depending on what's needed at the time. Insulin is indeed the body's principal fat-storage hormone. It asks fat cells to preserve food and avoids the decomposition of stored fat. When cells are (very common) insulin resistant, both sugar levels and insulin levels rise considerably. Chronically elevated rates of insulin (termed hyperinsulinemia) will contribute to multiple health problems, which include obesity and metabolic syndrome. Overeating — particularly sugar, refined carbohydrates, and fast food — continues to drive insulin resistance and raises insulin levels. Insulin is the body's primary fat-storage molecule. Reducing the intake of sugar, cutting carbohydrates, and workout are the best ways of reducing insulin levels.

Ghrelin

Ghrelin is known as a "hunger hormone." It releases ghrelin when your stomach is empty, which sends out a message to the hypothalamus telling you to eat. Normally, the levels of ghrelin are highest before eating, and the lowest about an hour after having a meal. Yet fasting ghrelin rates are also lower in overweight and obese people than in normal-weight men. Researches have shown that ghrelin only marginally reduces when obese individuals consume a meal. Just because of that, the hypothalamus is not getting a warning as good to avoid feeding, which may contribute to overeating. Eating plenty of protein and trying to avoid high sugar foods and drinks can help to optimize ghrelin levels.

Leptin

Leptin's made from your fat cells. It's called a "satiety hormone," reducing the hunger and making you feel whole. As an indicating hormone, its purpose is to communicate with the hypothalamus, the brain portion that regulates the intake of appetite and foods. Leptin informs the nervous system there is enough fat in storage and that there's no need for more, which helps to avoid overeating. People who are fat or overweight appear to have very large amounts of leptin in their plasma. In fact, one research concluded that leptin levels were 4 times higher in obese people than they were in normal-weight people. If leptin reduces appetite, then an obese person with greater leptin levels should begin to eat less and lose weight. Sadly the leptin mechanism isn't functioning as it should in obesity. This is termed resistance to leptin. When leptin signals are disrupted, the message to avoid eating does not go to the brain, and it doesn't know you've accumulated enough fat.

Your subconscious, in fact, feels it's hungry, and you're inclined to feed. Leptin levels are also lowered when you lose some weight, which is one of the main reasons why weight loss is so difficult to maintain in the long run. The brain believes you're hungry and tries to push you to consume enough. Chronically elevated levels of insulin and swelling in the hypothalamus are two possible causes of leptin resistance. Persons with obesity tend to resist leptin's effects. Eating anti-inflammatory foods, exercise regularly, and sleeping properly can improve the sensitivity to leptin.

Estrogen

Estrogen is the female sex hormone that is essential. It is produced primarily by ovaries and is involved in the regulation of the female reproductive system. Both extremely high and low estrogen rates may result in weight gain. That depends on age, other hormone action, and overall health status. Estrogen begins stimulating fat storage at puberty to preserve fertility all through reproductive years. It can enhance fat gain in the first half of pregnancy, in addition. Overweight women tend to have higher levels of estrogen than normal females, and some experts think this is due to environmental factors.

During menopause, the area for fat accumulation changes from the hips and thighs to visceral fat in the abdomen when estrogen levels drop because less is produced in the ovaries. This encourages insulin resistance and increases the risk of developing the disease. Such a way of life and diet approaches may assist with hormone control. If the estrogen levels are too high or too low, there may be weight gain. This is contingent on age and other hormonal influences.

Cortisol

Cortisol is a hormone that the adrenal glands make. It's defined as a "stress hormone" because when your body experiences stress, it is released. As with other hormones, survival is vital. Chronically elevated cortisol levels, however, can result in overeating and weight gain. Women who bear extra weight around the centre tend to react to distress with a significant rise in cortisol. But a restricted diet may also elevate cortisol. In one research, there were higher rates of cortisol among women who consumed a low-calorie diet and recorded feeling more depressed than women who eat regularly. High levels of cortisol will raise food consumption and lead to weight gain. Consuming a healthy diet, controlling tension, and getting sufficient sleep will help to stabilize the development of cortisol.

Glucagon-Like Peptide-1 (GLP-1)

Glucagon-like peptide-1 (GLP-1) is a hormone that is produced in your GI tract when nutrients enter the intestines. GLP-1 plays a major role in maintaining stable levels of blood sugar, and it also makes you feel full. Researchers claim the reduction in the desire to eat that occurs immediately after weight loss surgery is partly due to increased GLP-1 production. In one research, men who have been given a GLP-1 solution with breakfast felt physically more satisfied and ended up eating 12 percent lower calories at lunch. GLP-1 will lower appetite and promote weight loss. Consuming a high protein and green diet can help to increase your levels.

Neuropeptide Y (NPY)

Neuropeptide Y (NPY) is a hormone that cells within the brain and nervous system produce. It stimulates appetite, especially for refined carbs, and is the maximum all through time intervals of deprivation of food or fasting. Neuropeptide Y rates are increased during stressful cycles, which may contribute to an overheating and abdomen increase of weight. Neuropeptide Y (NPY) triggers hunger, especially during fasts and stressful times. Protein and soluble fibre can help to reduce NPY.

Peptide YY (PYY)

Another GI tract hormone that regulates the desire to eat is peptide YY (PYY). It is released into the digestive system and colon by cells. Peptide YY is thought to play an important part in decreasing food intake and reducing your risk of obesity. Start eliminating fried foods and consuming lots of fibre and protein to boost the PPY amounts and minimize hunger.

Cholecystokinin (CCK)

Like GLP-1, cholecystokinin (CCK) is another satiation hormone that the cells in your gut make. It has been demonstrated that higher levels of CCK decrease food intake in slim and fat people alike. CCK is an appetite-reducing hormone, generated when you consume protein, fat, and fibre.

Anything Else?

Hormones work together to promote or reduce appetite and store fat. If the mechanism is not working correctly, you might catch yourself continually battling with weight problems. Luckily, changes in diet and lifestyle may have strong effects on those hormones.

3.2 How your body fights weight loss?

And what makes It Want to Gain Weight Back.

Weight management is an essential part of a healthy life. Although many individuals effectively sustain healthier weights by a combination of diet and exercise, weight reduction may be critical to overweight or obesity-stricken 71 percent of Americans. But losing weight – especially extreme weight loss – is more difficult than eating fewer calories than burning. It would be won back by as much as 90 percent of individuals that have dropped substantial weight.

Sustainable weight management is achievable, and it will help you develop reasonable goals on your path to learning how the body reacts to weight reduction attempts.

Here are eight items you do not learn about body maintenance and weight loss.

Your Hormones Will Increase Drive to Eat

Sadly, caloric control is not the only method for the body to avoid weight loss, or to promote weight gain. Also at play are hunger hormones-leptin and ghrelin. Fat cells generate leptin, which informs the brain that it's complete. As you drop weight, the fat cells even decrease, releasing lesser leptin and ensuring you don't feel like a whole—1 strike. Ghrelin, made from the stomach, convinces the brain that it's time to resupply. The ghrelin rates increase as you lose weight, causing you to continue to consume more frequently. 2 Strike. Evidence shows that after a period of one year, neither leptin nor ghrelin rates rebound to a typical baseline.

Your Metabolic Rate Will Slow Down to Deposit Fat

The more you work out or control your calorie consumption to reduce weight, the more you tend to counteract your metabolism by speeding down to keep your existing weight— metabolic reinforcement steps in for potential energy recovery and fat conservation. Many doctors speculate this is how the human body has learned to prioritize food and energy preservation and to view a calorie deficit as a sign of suffering or famine.

Your Genes May or May Not Be Helpful

About 400 genes have been related to obesity and weight gain, which may influence eating, digestion, cravings, which distribution of body fat. The exact extent to which you may be genetically programmed to weight gain or obesity is uncertain, but genetic material has been correlated with increased loss difficulty even as you stay fit or diets with low calories. Like weight management in general, it is much easier to address a genetic predisposition for obesity from a preventive viewpoint than a reactionary one.

Your brain won't Remember How Much You're Eating.

The neuronal system of your brain, of contrast to your metabolism and hormones, is also battling weight loss. Food has a higher reward value after you lose weight as well as the area of the brain that controls food restriction becomes less effective – meaning that while you eat more to feel full (leptin's courtesy), you are less aware of how much you eat.

Your Body Is Prepared in Advance for Your Second Try

It creates antibodies to the disease when your body gets sick so that the immune system is ready the next time. Sadly it responds to weight loss in a similar manner. If you have lost weight in the past due to changes in exercise or diet and try to lose weight again with those same strategies, your body-again, mainly hormones, and metabolism-will modify to avoid additional damage, and you will see less weight loss results.

Your Weight Loss most probably will not look like what You Were Expecting

Unfortunately, after successful weight loss, it's not always smooth sailing anymore-especially successful extreme weight loss. Your body can look completely different from what you'd expected. Line marks and stretch marks are normal, and often people struggle with dealing with a body's internal consequences that don't seem like the dream they had in thought.

Your Weight Has a Favourite Number

Some researchers refer to the idea that your body has a fixed weight point, and all of this – your metabolic rate, hormone levels, Brain – will adjust to keep that weight going. The theory is that people can naturally have greater or lesser predefined weights than the others and genetics, aging, weight loss history, and other hormonal shifts can all have an impact on your set weight. In addition, set points may rise, but very seldom decrease. Likewise, they are also much better to sustain-as the body needs to-than to decrease, which is why it is simpler to retain a healthier weight than to lose weight.

Your Emotional Health Remains separate of Your Weight

As a consequence, people continue to tie pleasure and mental well-being to losing weight and slip into a spiral of disappointment because they have effectively lost weight but feel unhappy with certain facets of their lives. Besides the urge to binge and deal with these emotions, shame about not feeling satisfied following weight loss will also play about. In fact, certain people can feel confusion regarding what's next after losing large quantities of weight if it was their primary goal.

3.3 What Can Help

Some simple strategies can help support your weight loss goals, such as trying to make protein a mainstay of snacks and meals or begin a weight loss workout with cardio prior to actually swapping to lifting weights and resistance afterward. To work on their emotional well-being alongside weight loss, many people find it beneficial to focus on small, achievable lifestyle goals. Of starters, you may be focused on hitting a level where you feel confident playing a sport or taking a community workout class, rather than searching for a specific amount on the scale. Similarly, it can help you avoid the pitfalls of quick, short-term solutions by attempting for moderate aims that can eventually increase to bigger change.

Chapter 04: Hypnosis and Self-Hypnosis

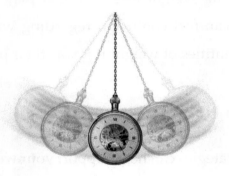

Hypnosis can be conducted by the professional, or you can also use the therapy all by yourself by just following the simple and basic steps which are discussed in detail in this chapter. Whether it's a self-hypnosis or hypnosis by a professional, it is beneficial for human health. Myths regarding hypnotherapy are also dismissed in this chapter so that one will be over any doubts regarding the therapy. Different factors triggering the overeating or emotional eating are discussed so that they can be overcome by the person and will not be a hindrance in losing weight

4.1 What is Self-Hypnosis?

Self-hypnosis-This carries some rather stupid interpretations. So this is not what self-hypnosis is, to clear these up:

• Self-hypnosis doesn't put a pendulum before your eyes.

• Self-hypnosis doesn't slip unconscious or into an involuntary trance from where it's hard to recover.

• Self-hypnosis doesn't lead to you losing control.

Conversely, self-hypnosis involves:

• Induce yourself to a highly suggestive state (this will be explored in the following).

• Full oversight and awareness of your actions.

• The freedom to leave your genetically modified mind condition anytime you wish.

Self-hypnosis basically involves inducing yourself into a very calm and amenable state of concentrated alertness. This increases the response of a person to suggestions, e.g., "I feel strong, confident and calm," "My body is totally relaxed and still," "I am free. I'm fine. Such suggestions are to be better reflected in the daily life of the person.

Nonetheless, self-hypnosis is such an effective technique that has been proven to successfully solve a variety of issues, including:

1. Matters of stress and anxiety.

2. Weight issues.

3. Chronic ache.

4. Depression.

5. Sleep disturbances.

6. Addictions.

7. Questions about self-esteem.

4.2 Steps to Enable Self-Hypnosis

• You would need to feel physically confident and secure to start the cycle. Seek to use a quick calming method.

• Choose an item on which you can concentrate your eyes and mind – hopefully, this item would include you gazing upward directly on the wall or ceiling in front of you.

• Free your mind of all thoughts and only concentrate on your goal. Obviously, this is hard to do, so take your time and let your emotions leave you.

• Become mindful of your pupils, talk of making your eyelids heavy, and shutting gradually. Concentrate on breathing while your eyes shut, breathe in a deep and even manner.

• Tell yourself every time you breathe out, you'll relax more. Slow your breathing, and let each breath relax deeper and deeper.

• Use your mind's eye to visualize a gentle movement of an object up and down or sideways. Maybe a metronome's hand or a pendulum-something that has a normal, long, yet steady movement. See the object sway back and forth in your mind's eye or up and down.

•Softly, gradually and monotonously start the countdown from ten in your mind, saying after each count, 10 I'm relaxing. '9 I'm calming etc.

• Believe, and remember that you will have reached your hypnotic state when you finish counting down.

•It is the time when you enter the hypnotic condition to reflect on the specific messages you've written. Focus on each statement-see it in the eye of your mind, repeat it in your thoughts. Relax and keep focused.

•Relax and clear your mind before getting out of your hypnotic state once again.

• Count steadily but energetically to 10. Reverse the process you used when you were counting down to your hypnotic state before. Use some positive messages, as you count, between every number. '1, I'll feel like I've had a full night' sleep when I wake up'... etc.

• When you hit 10 you feel fully awakened and reborn! Let your conscious mind slowly catch up with the day's events, and continue to feel refreshed.

4.3 Step-by-step Hypnotherapy for Weight Loss

Re-framing Your Food Addiction with Hypnosis

The first step to using weight loss hypnosis: recognizing why you are not attaining your objectives. How's this working out? A hypnotherapist will typically ask you questions about your weight loss, i.e., about your eating habits and exercise habits.

This gathering of information helps to identify what you might need to help with the work.

You would then be directed into an injection, a method of calming the body and mind and achieving a hypnosis state. Your subconscious is strongly suggestible whilst in hypnosis. You've lost the aware and rational mind – so the hypnotherapist will talk to the unconscious feelings explicitly.

The hypnotherapist may send you constructive feedback, affirmations in hypnosis, and can encourage you to imagine the improvements. With our multiple episodes of fat reduction hypnosis, you should seek this right now! Positive weight-loss hypnosis suggestions could include:

- Improving belief. Positive suggestions will strengthen your sense of confidence by encouraging language.

- Visualization of Success. You may be asked during hypnosis to envision having to meet your fitness goals and the way it leaves you feeling.

- Arranging that Inner Speech again. Hypnosis will help you control an inner voice that "doesn't want" to abandon junk food and transform it into a friend in the weight loss quest that is fast and more logical through constructive advice.

- Hitting the unconsciousness. In the hypnotic state, the implicit habits which contribute to unhealthy eating will begin to be recognized. In other words, you can become more aware of why we make unhealthy food choices and healthy eating and maintain more mindful food choices strategies.

- Fending off anxiety. Hypnotic suggestions can help tame your fear of failing to achieve weight loss. Fear is the number one reason people may not get started in the first place.

- Addressing and Reshaping Behavior Trends. Once you are in hypnosis, you can analyze and investigate how you use these instinctive reactions to eat, and "turn off." We can start slowing down by repetitive positive thinking and undoubtedly simply eliminate instant, involuntary consideration.

• Creating new modalities for coping. Hypnosis allows you to establish healthier ways to deal with stress, emotional

responses, and relationship issues. You might be asked to view a stressful situation, for example, and then envision yourself with a healthy snack to respond.

• Rehearsing Balanced Eating. You may be kept asking to improvise making healthy eating choices during hypnosis, i.e., being certain about taking food home at an eatery. This helps to make those healthier options easier. Rehearsal helps to control cravings, too.

• Making eating habits better. You may enjoy unhealthy foods and want them. Hypnosis can help you begin to establish a desire or inclination for healthy choices, which can also affect the portion sizes you select.

• Increasing Indicators of Unconscious. You might have mastered, by practice, to block out the messages that your body sends when you feel satiated. Hypnotherapy tends to help you to become more conscious of those metrics.

Naturally, not every suggestion applies to you. Your hypnotherapy program-whether you consult through a hypnotherapist or self-hypnosis-should include ideas specific to your food partnership.

Going to work with a licensed hypnotherapist may help you to analyze your strategies to address your specific needs.

4.4 How Hypnotherapy Helps You Achieve Weight Loss

In the hypnotic condition, the subconscious becomes much more accessible to persuasion. In reality, the study has also shown that during hypnotherapy, several remarkable improvements arise in the brain, which helps you to know without objectively worrying about the knowledge you are getting.

That is to say; you are separated from the skeptical mind. Therefore the vital rational mind does not doubt what you think when you seek hypnotic advice. And this, throughout a nutshell, is how hypnosis will help you knock down the obstacles stopping weight loss.

Persistence, however, is key to progress. That is why, after an initial session, many hypnotherapists send you off with self-hypnosis tapes. In your mind, the hurdles are strong. Only by continuous research will you untangle those assumptions effectively and reformulate them.

But hearing frequent statements and encouraging advice on balanced food is a first phase in the process towards weight loss. You're teaching people to think differently. Even those assumptions will support you:

Control Cravings

What if you can detach yourself from the cravings? Detach them and disperse them? Hypnosis methods for other weight reduction enable you to achieve so. For instance, you may be asked to imagine taking your cravings away – may be out to sea on a ship. Suggestions will also help you right-frame your cravings, and understand how to properly control them.

Expect Success

Perceptions determine truth. Naturally, since we have an anticipation of achievement, we are more likely to take the requisite measures to reach that performance. Hypnotherapy for weight loss can sow the seeds of achievement in your subconscious, which may be a potent unconscious motivator to keep you on course.

Practice Positivity

Negativity so often spoils weight loss. There are things which you can't eat. Unhealthy food "kills" you. Hypnotherapy allows us to re-frame these ideas in a more positive light-you don't starve yourself; you lose what you don't need.

Prepare for Relapse

We've been trained to think there are humiliating relapses – excuses to give up. Yet hypnosis tells one to talk differently about a relapse. A relapse is a chance to analyze what went wrong, benefit from it, and be more equipped to be tempted.

Modify Your Behavior

One little step at a time meets major objectives. Hypnotherapy encourages us to make small changes that feed into larger objectives. Tell you're rewarding yourself with high sugar, high-calorie foods; you may be focusing on finding a healthy incentive by hypnosis.

Visualize Success

Hypnotic vision, finally, is a strong motivator. Visualization allows you to "sense" consequences and discuss how they make you feel. You could also visualize your future-self, saying you have what it takes to succeed.

4.5 Self-Hypnosis for Releasing Bad Eating Habits: What You Will Do

When it comes to hypnotherapy, individuals have a few options: one-on-one meetings with a hypnotherapist, listening to tapes of hypnosis, and self-hypnosis. Self-hypnosis is among the most useful, as you can do it at home or at the

workplace.

Meat addictions are also highly recommended. As you can see, that is a simple process. Here are a few points you might want to keep in mind:

• Notice the Wellness: How do you feel? Assessing how you felt is good, and by the conclusion of the session, you will reassess it.

• Directed meditation and visualization: deep breathing shows that recovery is available for the body and mind. Visualization is also another form of calming initiation.

• A Directed Countdown: You will count down from 10. This helps the mind enter a hypnosis-state.

• Positive Assertions: You can directly communicate to the subconscious once you're relaxed. Offer affirmations to it, positive suggestions for reconditioning the mind. For food abuse, for instance, you could say things like: "I'm safe from overeating. I listen to know my body when to eat. I like to consume full servings of nutritious foods. I'm stopping sugary foods. Every single day, I feel better.

• Visualizing the Change: Imagine how you'll pursue the safer direction once you've offered your subconscious constructive feedback. See yourself living in a healthy food relationship.

This strengthens the idea and allows it to take hold and to sustain it.

4.6 Who should try hypnosis?

The best client, frankly, is someone who has difficulty committing to a balanced diet and fitness routine because their bad patterns don't want to lift. It's a symptom of a subconscious issue to get caught in harmful habits — like eating the whole bag of potato chips instead of quitting when you're finished.

Your subconscious is the position where the thoughts, patterns, and addictions reside. And since hypnotherapy is treating the subconscious, rather than only the aware, it may be more successful. Nevertheless, a 1970 research report showed that hypnosis has a success rate of 93 percent, with fewer treatments available for both psychotherapy and behavioral counseling. "This led researchers to believe that hypnosis was the most effective method for changing habits, thought patterns, and behavior.

And could hypnotherapy be used on its own? Hypnosis can also be used as a complement to other weight loss programs developed by physicians to manage different conditions of

well-being, be it diabetes, hypertension, asthma, or cardiovascular diseases.

4.7 Does hypnotherapy work for weight loss?

Hypnosis can be more successful for those trying to lose weight than diet and exercise alone. The aim is to be able to manipulate the mind and alter behaviors like overeating. Nonetheless, it's always up for discussion just how powerful it can be.

An earlier, controlled trial examined the use of hypnotherapy in people with obstructive sleep apnea for weight loss. The research explored two different types of hypnotherapy and basic nutritional recommendations for weight loss and sleep apnea. Within three months, all 60 participants lost 2 to 3 percent of their body weight.

The hypnotherapy participant had shed, on average, an additional 8 pounds at the 18-month follow-up. While this additional loss was not significant, the researchers concluded that hypnotherapy justified more studies as a treatment for obesity.

A weight-reduction study that involved hypnotherapy, primarily cognitive-behavioral therapy (CBT), found that this

culminated in a slight drop in body weight relative to the placebo community. Researchers have hypothesized that although hypnotherapy can improve weight loss, there is not enough work to persuade them.

It's important to remember that there is not any evidence for weight reduction in favor of hypnosis alone. Most of what you'll learn in conjunction with food and exercise or treatment is in hypnotherapy.

4.8 Stop Emotional Eating: Subliminal Hypnosis

What Triggers Emotional Eating?

To live, we need food. That's not necessarily the explanation we cook, however. The emotional eating cause would most definitely be unique for every person, but there are certain specific feelings that activate emotional eating – that is, feeding not to relieve hunger but to provide immediate relief from stressful feelings. That's this depressed eating trend that contributes to poor eating patterns and resulting weight gain. Typical emotional-eating causes are:

• Blame.

• Poor self-esteem

• The feeling of continuous failure

• The Solitude

• Stress

• Frustration

• Anxiety

The greatest misconception is this – the aforementioned feelings cause emotional eating, but the shame and long-term weight gain arising from emotional eating will tend to activate certain feelings all over again! Instead, then grappling with anger by confronting the root-mental eaters, then head for the fridge and eventually wind up becoming worse.

The Painful Cycle of Emotional Eating

We've learned that people don't eat only to relieve hunger. Emotional feeding focuses on utilizing words and connections. We can let one thing stand for another that normally serves our race well in introducing new processes and pretty advanced culture. However, we use affiliation and representations very much in a derogatory way. They may also equate a particular pang of guilt with a pang of hunger as referring to emotional feeding. So it is a normal belief under these situations that feeding would fix the problem.

Then why do we name emotional eating a loop? Because its negative feelings of shame that fill up in after we eat, trigger much of the same thoughts and emotions and start the cycle again. That behavior isn't really deliberate; this just tends to happen. We have trained ourselves in such a way that it is hard to alter. Ever wondered why a dog would get enthused when he senses the tinkering tone in the kitchen? He connects the sound by making him served a meal. The term 'classical conditioning' refers to this type of association.

4.9 Hypnotherapy Can Aid You to Change Developed Habits through the Power of Hypnosis

Crack the cycle of comfort eating by resolving the issue at the point that it is rooted in the unconscious mind. You can see some important improvements take place over the process of hypnotherapy treatment:

• You're becoming more comfortable and your thinking is simpler

• Holding the emotional and social needs apart will start to sound normal and therefore inevitably happen

• You should search for more innovative ways to channel the thoughts and work with them

- The appetite for healthier food will increase and it will significantly boost the diet

- You will continue to feel more optimistic, more comfortable, and satisfied with your everyday life without a relentless cross.

4.10 Health Benefits of Hypnosis

No longer to over-eat

Seeking to make healthier choices and getting exercise are major elements of losing weight, but an effective fat loss in some instances also necessitates steering clear of sentimental and unintentional barriers that inhibit us from weight loss. Using hypnotherapy for losing weight takes a comprehensive approach than if used for other health problems — it typically takes numerous meetings to evaluate the personal triggers of the person, rather than just one. Before hypnotherapy is conducted, the expert needs to discover out whether they are all-day snackers and those who reach between meals in the refrigerator. Everyone is special, everybody can have their own addiction, so figuring it out requires a little while. You shut your eyes after five to six bites and remind yourself, 'that's enough,' so if you consume a bowl of food, you shut your eyes and suggest 'eat about half of what's in it.'

Cure phobia within the dental profession

The drill's high-pitched whirl, the needle poke, or the humiliation by making somebody peek into your mouth are only a couple of the reasons people stop visiting the dentist. Although the industry is trying to utilize modern dental technologies to render a ride to the dentist's office less painful, dental discomfort affects between 10 to 20 percent of the world's population. Fear has, for years, driven several of my patients from the dentist seat. Fear can originate from a traumatic dental encounter or learning from someone that has had a bad experience. Whatever the case, it may be debilitating because if it's conditioned, the subconscious will work in the default setting. To help clients overcome the discomfort about going to the dentist, neuro-linguistic programming (NLP) is used that lets the brain "rewire" those thinking patterns to get past loops of negative thinking. NLP may be used to stop the fear and rewire the phobia to their own as they continue to experience fear regarding visiting the dentist.

Maintain grief

Whether it is coping with a national disaster or a loved one's death, it may undermine the sense of grief or bereavement, triggering fear, insomnia, and depression. Letting yourself experience the pain by grieving improves your body and mind, like learning about your loved one's passing, taking care of your well-being, reaching out to those who have to cope with the tragedy, acknowledging your emotions and living the existence of the one you missed. The strategies to cope with the loss are psychological. Hypnotherapy can assist by offering constructive feedback to help deal with mourning feelings and help discover solutions to live with the suffering as time passes on. Professionals are helping people deal with suffering by setting a "timer" on grief and loss. "Normally, when they're tired and emotionally exhausted and tired of grieving, they let the professional knowledge.

Detain tinnitus

As per the American Tinnitus Association, ticking, clicking, hissing, whooshing, or whistling noises that no one except you can hear are symptoms of tinnitus, a disease that 45 million Americans endure. Though hearing loss may be acute or continuous, most forms of the disorder may not obtain the cure. Treatment methods include hearing aids, behavioral counseling, sound therapy, and TMJ. Hypnosis is an alternative, as well. "The mindset induces tinnitus; it tends to actually occur because the person expects that to happen, and the sound disappears even after you disable the idea of anticipating it.

More tolerable Chemotherapy

Some of the first known examples of cancer patient hypnosis were in 1829 when M. Le Docteur Chapelain utilized hypnosis to alleviate breast cancer patients' pain. During a mastectomy, the doctor utilized hypnotherapy as a general anesthetic, and the woman was reported to be "calm and displayed excellent pain control" during the surgery. Although anesthesia is the favored method for surgery today, hypnosis often plays a part in cancer care and is sometimes used to relieve discomfort and distress as well as alleviate the side effects of treatment like vomiting and diarrhea. They help them mainly cope with the effects and help them improve how they handle stress. The therapist won't give them false optimism, but they place them in a safe position to help them recover. Cancer victims are sometimes moved from hospital to hospital, allowing them to feel as though they're only a few. Therapists make unique tapes to which the patients listen during their procedure with treatment — it's a real interaction with a hypnotherapist that could go afar.

Boost efficiency in athletics

Michael Jordan, Tiger Woods, and Mike Tyson are really just a few other well-known elite athletes who have transformed into hypnotherapy to support their performance in athletics. Athletes have often utilized hypnotherapy to remove stressful emotions, de-stress and calm the mind and body, and assist in improving attention and relaxation so that they might "be in the zone." This behavioral stimulation will enhance motivation, performance, and skill and extends to all types of performers, including those suffering from trauma and those only starting a sport. Many players go through a hypnotist to enhance their output when, in essence, they're trying to strengthen their minds. A hypnotist will transform the thought mechanism to convert negative behaviors into good ones. It requires a lot of cognitive toughness to be a productive golfer. 'You've got to adjust the understanding to experience, so you've got to approach the game psychologically like w.

Faster recuperation from the operation

Hypnosis is used to support post-surgery patients reduce their healing period and, in some situations, wean them off medication administered by the doctor. Thoughts and feelings flow through paths, so that's how patterns are formed. At first, it's only a route through the trees, so with the period the road gradually is becoming a pit, you can't get out of. Through hypnosis, the nervous system and brain are guided to take a different pathway.

Symptoms of Irritable Bowel Syndrome (IBS)

Scientific research has generally confirmed the effects of hypnosis on IBS. IBS is stomach pressure produced by the bowels, so hypnosis may help relieve symptoms like constipation, vomiting, so bloating. Often IBS may trigger other symptoms, such as nausea, exhaustion, back pain, and urinary issues.

How it tends to work: Hypnosis takes you into gradual recovery, offering calming thoughts and stimuli to combat the effects you encounter.

Weight Loss

Like with the prevention of smoking, there are currently not enough trials that would validate the efficacy of weight reduction hypnosis, while several researchers have observed moderate weight loss — around 6 pounds during 18 months — by hypnosis. If hypnosis has been used in conjunction with improvements in exercise and diet, it is typically most effective.

How it tends to work: When you're hypnotized, the emphasis is on the mind. This helps you more inclined to react and react to recommendations about improvements in your lifestyle, such as following a healthier diet or exercising regularly, which may promote weight loss.

Quit Cigarette Smoking

Cigarettes are not easy to give up. There are other ways to support you leave, such as prescribed drugs or the nicotine patch. Although the study is still around, several individuals have considered hypnosis to have enabled them to quit the problem of smoking.

Smoking reduction hypnosis performs better while you are practicing one-on-one with a hypnotist who will tailor the hypnosis treatments to fit the lifestyle.

How it tends to work: You need to really want to stop smoking in an attempt for hypnosis to function for quitting smoking. Hypnotherapy may be used in two forms. One of which is to help you identify a safe, successful alternative practice and then direct your subconscious toward the behavior instead of smoking. This could be like munching a stick of gum or going for a walk. The second is to prepare the subconscious to equate cigarettes with unpleasant stimuli, such as a bitter aftertaste in the mouth or a disgusting scent of smoke.

Anxiety

Relaxation methods — hypnosis including — will also relieve fear. Hypnosis appears to be most successful in patients whose distress is triggered by a specific disorder of well-being — such as cardiac failure — rather than generalized fear.

Hypnosis can also benefit if you are dealing with a phobia — a form of anxiety condition where you are deeply scared about something that doesn't pose a major danger.

How it helps: Hypnosis helps to relieve fear by stimulating the body to trigger its normal reaction to stimulation through utilizing an expression or nonverbal signal, slowing down breathing, reducing blood pressure, and trying to instill an improved feeling of well-being.

Problematic Sleep, Sleepwalking, and Insomnia

Hypnotherapy can be a valuable method whether you're sleepwalking or trying to fall and remain asleep. Hypnosis will calm you enough to allow you to sleep better if you have insomnia.

Hypnosis will also teach you to wake up anytime you hear your feet touch the floor to help you stop sleepwalking trysts, whether you're a sleepwalker.

And if you can only need to have a little more night, hypnosis will even assist with that. Learning the methods of self-hypnosis will improve the period of time you rest and the period of time you spend in deep sleep — the sort of sleep you need to wake up and feel refreshed.

How it works: visual signals place you in a trance-like environment, close to how you experience when you're so absorbed in a book or video that you don't realize what's happening around you. You'll fall asleep during hypnosis — or just after that —.

Severe Pain

Hypnosis may assist relieve pain — such as during surgery, migraine headaches, or seizures with stress. And persistent depression can improve, too. Individuals with pain associated with conditions such as asthma, cancer, sickle cell anemia, and fibromyalgia — as well as people with lower back pain — can receive hypnosis relief.

Why it works: Hypnosis will allow you to deal with pain and develop more self-control regarding suffering. However, findings show that hypnosis over extended stretches of time will achieve so successfully.

Chapter 05: Meditation

This chapter discusses in detail all the aspects of meditation and its role in the well-being of human health that how it brings the body and mind in harmony and helps them to function accordingly and healthily. Several health benefits of meditation are also discussed in detail so that the person opting for it will not have any doubt regarding its effectiveness and health benefits. It is also explained how it will be beneficial in reducing the weight if exercise and changed eating patterns tend to fail in order to do so.

5.1 What is meditation?

Meditation is a practice that actually brings the mind and body together to achieve a sense of calm. People meditated as a personal activity for thousands of years. Today, many people are using meditation to relieve tension and become more mindful of their feelings. There are many different kinds of meditation. Many are focused on the usage of such words or mantras. Others, in the current moment, rely on breathing or holding the mind. Both of these approaches will help you recognize yourself deeper and how the mind-body functions.

This enhanced sensitivity allows exercise a helpful method to grasp your food patterns deeper and may contribute to weight loss.

What's the connection between weight loss and meditation?

Meditation may be an important tool for helping individuals shed pounds. In that regard, what exactly makes meditation so effective? This aligns the conscious and unconscious mind by deciding to improvements to our actions that we choose to implement. Those improvements may involve managing excessive food cravings and changing eating habits. It is necessary to include the unconscious mind as this is where unhealthy, weight-gaining habits like emotional eating are rooted. Meditation will help you become more mindful of these and circumvent them with exercise, and also substitute them with weight loss practices.

Yet meditating provides a more immediate reward. Meditation may bring down the rates of stress hormones directly. Stress hormones like cortisol send our bodies a signal to preserve calories as fat. When you have a lot of adrenaline running into your body, even though you make good decisions, it's going to be difficult to lose some weight! We know it sounds hard; we're both stressed out, so shaking seems unlikely. Yet what it takes to substantially relieve depression is 25 minutes of meditation three days in a row.

With everyday practice, your self-control might also increase. The brain sections most influenced by meditation have become those that allow us to regulate ourselves. That means a few minutes of regular meditation will make things easier to pass on the second cookie or resist the ice cream when you feel low.

Understanding the terminology around meditation for weight loss

Different activities and methods — meditation, mindful eating, and intuitive feeding — may help us understand or relearn how to establish a balanced food partnership and how to avoid any negative cooking thoughts we might have. Weight reduction can be a side effect of maintaining this revived partnership, but the primary aim is not to create weight loss. Using this will constrain us so that we can't really feed intuitively or attentively.

Rather, concentrate on enjoying food — feeding when you're happy, not because you're depressed, and feeling frustrated with work or family problems. Through these practices, you'll understand and appreciate and love your body for everything it can do for you.

If it comes to talking weight loss meditation or eating meditation and moving on maintaining a healthier interaction with food, it will help to clarify what the dialect entails.

Mindful eating is a strategy or process that may be utilized to better fix diet and nutrition interactions in your association. It requires us to be conscious and to interact with our senses — how the food looks, feels, and, most significantly, how everything makes our bodies sound. Cautious eating includes intuitive eating, making us calm down and listening to our inner signals of real appetite and signals of satiation, which as such, will help us decrease or even fully avoid our mental or binge eating. While mindful eating will contribute to weight loss, the aim or inspiration should not be to lose weight. If our meal choices are made predicated on that physical outcome that we desire, it implies that we have stopped eating intently already.

Anxiety or emotional eating happens when, because of intense emotions or thoughts, individuals choose to consume and overeat rather than respond to their own internal hunger signals. Such thoughts will also overshadow our actual sensations of contentment and satiety while we encounter intense emotions, and that may lead to us over-eating. Food is seen as a calming strategy in such situations, temporarily masking intense feelings. Recognizing that such experience contributes to the perpetuation of a cycle is essential, though. Having unpleasant feelings may contribute to binge consumption, contributing to remorse or embarrassment, going back to feeling — and not able to tolerate or manage — negative emotions or anxiety.

Intuitive eating is a mind-body strategy for health and well-being, which is not a diet. It opposes the diet idea and encourages us to trust our bodies and respond to our internal physical signs in order to restore our food relationship. Intuitive feeding contains concepts of healthy cooking. However, it also requires a wider extended concept that stretches throughout, pushing the body as it feels nice to walk, and use dietary knowledge without discrimination.

5.2 How can meditation help when diet and exercise don't seem to be working?

Stress is a key cause in certain situations for unhealthy weight gain or the failure to lose weight effectively. And, if you've been counting calories and exercising but are still depressed, the issue that holds the weight on may not be solved. Stress again activates hormones that store excess fat — exactly what we don't want. It can also intensify a tension cycle: You can't lose weight when you're stressing out, which leaves you upset because you can't lose weight. Becoming trapped in is a simple cycle, but you can escape it-and meditation will aid.

To deal with or eliminate stress better, first you need to understand what causes most of it in your life. Some stressors may be quickly recognized, but some may be subtler.

5.3 How to Meditate?

Many forms to meditate. The CDC notes that these four items are typical to certain forms of meditation:

• **Silent spot.** You should pick your perfect chair-where to meditate. On a trek? This is about you.

• **A specific relaxed pose,** such as sitting, lying, standing, or walking.

• **Focus center.** You should focus on one term or expression, the breath, or something else.

• **Free mindedness.** Having other thoughts whilst you are meditating is normal. Attempt not to venture into those feelings too often. Continue to bring your focus back to your breath, series of words, or whatever else you are focusing on.

Pick the location, period, and process you'd like to try. You should even join a class to understand the fundamentals.

What are the benefits of meditation for weight loss?

Meditation is not going to help you lose weight immediately. Yet with a little preparation, it will actually have lifelong impacts not just on your weight but also on your ways of thought.

Sustainable weight loss

Meditation provides a number of aspects to practice. Mindfulness therapy appears to be the most effective in terms of weight reduction. A review of existing research in 2017 found that meditation on mindfulness was an effective method for weight loss and changing eating habits.

The reflection on carefulness requires paying very close attention to:

• Whereabouts

• What you're up to

• How you are feeling right now

Throughout contemplation on mindfulness, you can remember all these things without judgment. Try to treat your thoughts and actions just like those — none other. Take control of what you expect and experience, but don't try to label something as positive or negative. Through routine practice, that becomes simpler.

Practicing meditation with consciousness can also offer long-term benefits. Many that practice exercise is more likely to hold off the weight compared with other dieters.

Less guilt and shame

Meditation is mindfulness may be a great benefit in curtailing mental and stress-related consumption. You will notice the moments that you feed when you're nervous, rather than starving, by being more conscious of your feelings and emotions.

It's also a helpful way to stop from slipping down the dangerous trap of embarrassment and remorse that other people are sliding through while attempting to improve their eating behaviors. Meditation of mindfulness requires acknowledging the thoughts and actions for what they are, without criticizing yourself.

It helps you to excuse yourself for committing mistakes, including consuming a bag of potato chips for starters. The forgiving will also keep you from becoming tragic, which is a sophisticated word for what occurs when you want to buy a pizza, and by consuming a bag of chips, you've already "messed things up."

Chapter 06: Affirmation and Mantras

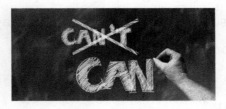

Different types of affirmations for different occasions are discussed in this chapter so as to achieve the target. Mantras that date back to ancient times also have healing powers and a positive impact on the human body. Mantras are the chants used repeatedly to bring the mind and body in synchronization. Although both terms are used interchangeably, there are still major differences between the two. How the affirmations are practiced and how they are helpful for different purposes is discussed in this chapter. Affirmation for a positive mind set, body image, and self-control are discussed in detail.

6.1 What Are Positive Affirmations?

Positive affirmations are positive statements describing a desired outcome, routine, or goal you wish to achieve. Repeating these positive statements often affects the subconscious mind deeply, and stimulates it into action, bringing into real life what you are parroting.

The act of mentally or loudly repeating the affirmations motivates the individual to repeat them, enhances confidence and inspiration, and creates incentives for change and success.

This act also programs the mind to act in accordance with repeated words, sparking the subconscious mind to work on one's behalf, making the factual claims come to fruition.

• Affirmations are really helpful in creating healthy routines, achieving meaningful improvements in one's life, and attaining goals.

• The affirmations help to lose weight, to become more centred, to learn more, to improve behaviours, and to fulfil goals.

• They may be useful in athletics, industry, health-enhancing, bodybuilding, and many other fields.

• These positive statements affect the body, the mind and one's feelings in a favourable way

It is very normal to repeat affirmations, but most individuals are not conscious of this. People often echo pessimistic, not constructive proclamations. This is known as negative self-talk.

When you tell yourself how miserable you are, how inadequate to learn, have not enough resources, or how tough life is, you reinforced pessimistic affirmations.

In this way, you generate more difficulties and many more issues because you focus on the troubles, and therefore increase them, rather than concentrating on the solutions.

Most people repeat negative words and statements in their minds about the unpleasant experiences and situations in life and thus create more unwanted situations.

Words work to build or demolish in both ways. It is the manner we utilize them that decides how they can produce positive or negative outcomes.

6.2 Do affirmation work?

There might be scepticism about this topic, especially since motivational phrases are often provided as wondrous but under a more divine light, in which we are probably not identifying ourselves.

Reiterating the same sentences multiple times can not appear to be the most exciting thing to do, and might even sound tedious.

But are you risking something, if you attempt it? You are the only one who has direct exposure to the inside of your head, and no one else knows what happens inside it if you either repeat some positive affirmations or if your parts of the brain have chosen to go to the beach.

Positive affirmations which work, but don't make miracles

Compelling affirmations don't perform magic, and they don't add miracles to our lives just by attempting to read them for several days. However, they can be quite advantageous if used to accomplish our changes/goals in accordance with the approved behaviour chosen.

For instance, if you reiterate to yourself that the only meal I want is nutritious food, my behaviour will have to go along, that is, I will try whatever I can to stop taking some fast food home and simply avoid purchasing it.

Another reason is that if we say many times per day that we are indeed a good individual then stick on the same behaviours as normal, it would be really unlikely for us to lose weight, gain strength or grow stronger.

6.3 Use of positive affirmations

Here are a few guiding principles for utilizing optimistic affirmations to more effectively shed weight:

1. Release your attachment to limiting beliefs.

You may have beliefs about why you think you can't lift the weight. Such assumptions that emerge from negative reminders from adolescence, such as, "You can never contribute to something" or naive compliance with social thinking, such as, "Everybody thinks it's hard to lose weight." Make space for optimistic affirmations to take root by changing your mind to replacing perceptions that hinder you with uplifting values that help you. Using this fast test method to assess if a belief is supporting you or harming you:

"Will the belief generate fear or doubt?

"Is this belief contrary to my ambitions?

If perception does not back you up, adjust it.

2. Create affirmations that feel natural to you.

If you trust in them, the strength of affirmations grows, because they become important. However, even though it doesn't sound real yet, you may use affirmations to step slowly in the direction of who you want to become. For example, if you say, "I release weight easily" but underneath it all, you don't believe that, create an affirmation that feels truly like, "I'm open to lifting weight with greater ease," or, "I'm capable of achieving my goals even though this sometimes feels difficult."

3. Use "I Am" statements whenever possible.

"I am" statements are particularly powerful because we become whatever we attach to the words, "I am." Inside us, there is a spiritual force, and it pays special attention to whatever follows our statements about "I am." And if you're thinking, "I'm a loser," or "I'm a winner," you're triggering a strong performance that works.

Use "I am" statements to reflect the qualities that you want, even though they don't seem true yet. When you interact with the positive energies within you, your declarations regarding "I am" will deliver the outcomes you want in time.

4. Say affirmations in the present tense.

The world listens quite simply to the feelings and opinions and reacts in response. Create affirmations that will serve you at this moment and not at some future date.

For starters, if you think, "I'm trying to lose weight," it leaves your progress stagnant for an undetermined future. Yet if you claim, "I'm losing weight," you're already affirming improvement.

5. Use affirmations when you feel relaxed and peaceful.

Once we are in a relaxed environment, affirmations enter our subconscious mind more quickly. While repeating affirmations throughout the day is important, it also creates some quiet time to deepen its effects.

A Daily Practice

• Choose from a list of two or three affirmations. Adjust them to fit you better, or create your own.

• Say your statements three to five times, or more, all day long.

• Write them on 35 cards to take with you, apply them to the backdrop of your screen, or write them on post-it notes located in noticeable places such as your bathroom mirror or vehicle.

• Create a quiet time during the day when you can sit back and repeat them peacefully.

• Say your affirmations with a profound feeling, as when you already acquire the qualities that you assert.

6.4 Sample Affirmations

• "I'm able to send up weight now."

• "I deserve perfect health now, and accept it."

• "They respect me."

• "I'm in good health."

- "I love my body and accept it as I release weight for my better health and happiness."

- "I can quickly release weight."

- "I listen to what my body requires of me."

- "I am affectionate with myself and others, and I forgive."

- "I feel diligent with my body and myself."

- "I'm changing my lifestyle to a healthy way of life."

6.5 The 10 Affirmations to love your body

I am sound and lean

A first is a faith in your physique. You are in the "I would like to be healthful and lean," space. I really want that. Declaring it now as your reality, "I'm safe and lean," lets the body take mostly on strength. When you assert it and the area of learning, and enjoy it emotionally by feeling positive about the reality which is your true strength. If it weren't true, then you would be absolutely satisfied where you will be.

Your present state tells me this is accurate, because you're discontented. If you want the facts to materialize today, and you can say realities as though they are now your reality and you are generating it as you do. I am lean and healthy. Allow it the basis of your own self-esteem. It is your body that wants to own it. That has the entire capability to build a lean, balanced environment. It needs to be lean and healthy. Believe in the flesh.

I consider myself outside food

I remember myself, above the rice. So much do you consider yourself as the incentive, and use food? Hey, I am feeling guilty too. Also, some other day I spotted myself being, "Ah, I'm that way, you understand, I really feel excited. I just finished this. I'll give me something nice to eat. "I believe it links that down to our upbringing as adolescents where food also used a little to seek to evoke social cooperation. "They're getting paid. Let me award you here." Navigating as a mom is a profoundly difficult activity not to use nutrition as an incentive. "You could have a dessert, yes. Just you consume this because ... "the trend persists as we are using meal as a means to remember oneself. That sends us down. Because we are happier to consume junk food, because so we use meals as acceptance, such as the baked goods that are actually enjoyable to the container.

I'm Loving My Body

But, you are going to go further than that. I remember myself, above the rice. I love myself and weight just vanishes. Let it speak for yourself. Knew that the body responds to oneself? Are you indignant? Would you even say that you hate your own body? Look into a mirror, and bring it aside, would you tell a good friend you respect and adore the needs you think to your body? Your body only responds to you. The fat cells react. You're going. "Well I guess I'm going to react accordingly." Learn to respect your skin now.

In our knowledge, we have this groovy thing with when we choose to respect and cherish our brain in a scenario we don't want, we assume we choose to allow it, like, "Oh, I don't care. I'm indifferent and now I really love my body. I don't mind it ever changing. "No! It is the most exalted sound to elicit shift. When you feel good, the body is inspired to make a difference. If your body is feeling shameful and trying to run shameful energy, it needs to go eat junk. Healthier options won't support it. He's not likely to feel like running. Loving will trigger improvement for you. I hated my girlfriend and

weight just vanishes.

I Am My Real Power

Catch oneself, then. Look into a mirror or then go "What do you know? That's about the reason it is. I will want to adore it correctly now. "I will use affection as a tool of assistance to evoke transformation in my stomach. I am my perfect weight. "Ok, hey, because you're in the room, you're trying to throw in," Eh, that's not real. "You've got to build for a conviction what you desire first. Then assume it, and you will see it.

In my dresses I feel great

I look good in my shoes. That is a tough one because while you're not in the height, it's also hard to look comfortable in your shoes, you are not the weight you want to be in the amount you'd like. I have a wonderful plan in order to support you through this. Right now, today, I can make you relax great in your clothes, no matter what size or shape. You want to start feeling wonderful in your dresses and proclaim that as one's truth and in my clothes feel great. They're trying to build it.

I will be saying "no" to stuff that doesn't keep me happy

How much food should you answer yes with that's not a healthy pattern for you? How if you'd only been collected to tell no quickly? Easily argue no to types of food you don't think are healthy. This creed will inspire you to pick. Avoid pouring money into poor food options, and then create proclamations.

I am fascinated by my body by resources and food

So, we've got a sort of duality here. I'll say no to it and I'm really derived from that now. Yeah, draw ...... it feels yeah ... I feel pushed. I feel very easily involved with it. It is rather effortless than, "Oh, I've got to eat it. I live in poverty. I don't want to do this. "You would like to feel loved; you're fascinated by it. I 'm drawn by the resources and food my body supports. I'm made of proclamations that mask my body's discomfort.

I 'm happy with the correct quantity of food

I really love it though. So far less can you feed on holding your belief? I have had enough of that. My desire is full. I am finished. I feel happy.

I don't need to have excess weight to cover me

All correct. This gets serious. So, this is, "Whoa, this got a little bit of heavy duty." Got several other stuff is going to support you on this and only say it's the reality when you're, like, "Whoa, you know, for some purpose I need some security from the universe." Okay, I've got some resources that'll really support you fix some. You know, then, as a shielded barrier, you don't need weight.

I look into a mirror and look just how I enjoy a safe and balanced body

So now, when you actually try to do this as I look into a mirror, I have seen a safe, athletic body which I enjoy. Will you see the organism that needs to express itself for sure? The organ that needs to live up to it? The organ that needs to reveal yourself? Could you glance at your present life in the reflection and look the future in there? Using this move. He. He. What's the look like? How would you feel like on the legs? Your chest, muscles in it? What does that make you feel? Think as it's occurring right now. Give yourself love and don't presume to receive it from some other men.

6.6 Self-control affirmations

What Is Self-Control?

People frequently use a wide range of self-control terms, including restraint, perseverance, grit, willpower, and fortitude.

Usually, psychologists describe self-regulation as:

- The desire to monitor behavior, to resist temptations and accomplish goals

- The capacity to withhold gratification and to tolerate unhealthy actions or impulses

- A resource small, which can be diminished

Currently, some scholars suggest that biology partially dictates self-control, with some only born smarter than others.

Why self-control is important for well-being?

Self-control is the capacity to monitor and modify actions to prevent negative activities, improve beneficial habits, and accomplish long-term objectives. Evidence has shown that maintaining self-control may be vital for well-being and well-being. Popular resolutions such as weight reduction, daily workout, healthier living, not fretting, surrendering unhealthy behavior, and saving the money are only a few worthy aspirations people feel require self-control.

Importance

If the aim is to shed pounds, graduate from college, or stop smoking, it's tempting to assume that reaching a target is just a question of managing the habits. Many people surveyed agree that self-control can be established, as well as improved.

Studies have often established different causes and approaches that may help individuals strengthen their self-control.

Researchers found that people with stronger self-control tend to live healthier and happier than others.

Students who displayed more self-discipline in one trial received improved marks; higher examination results were more likely to be accepted to a successful university program. The research also showed that self-control was a much more significant aspect than the Intelligence scores when it comes to academic achievement.

Self-control effects aren't restricted to educational outcomes. One long-term health study suggested that participants who were given good self-control rates during early life tended to have high levels of adult physical and mental health.

Delaying Gratification

An essential aspect of self-control is the desire to prolong the excitement or hesitate to get what you want. Individuals are also able to regulate their actions by suppressing their need for gratification. For example, a person adopting a specific diet might be attempting to escape the urges of wallowing in junk products. This person delays their enjoyment and awaits until they can appreciate an occasional treat.

Delaying satisfaction requires offsetting short-term expectations with long-term benefits. Studies also have shown that the capacity to postpone gratification is not just essential for meeting objectives but also serves a significant role in well-being and general life performance.

The Marshmallow Test

In the 1970s the psychologist Walter Mischel performed a number of popular studies exploring the value of delayed gratification. Children were offered a choice in these experiments: they could choose to eat one treat straight away (generally a candy bar or a marshmallow), or they might wait a limited period to get two treats. The researcher will then leave a child alone in a room with a single reward at this stage.

Not unexpectedly, the moment researchers left the room, several of the children opted to consume the single treat. Some of the other kids could wait until the second reward, though.

Researchers observed that children that were willing to defer gratification in order to obtain a higher incentive were often more likely to have improved academic results than those children that automatically ceded to pressure.

The "Hot-and-Cool" System

Based on his work, Mischel developed what he termed a "hot-and-cool" method to illustrate how satisfaction might be postponed. The hot mechanism applies to the mental, impulsive component of our determination and encourages us to perform on our wishes. When this mechanism takes control, we can give in to our current impulses and behave rashly without taking into consideration the likely long-term consequences.

The cool mechanism is the logical, reflective component of our willpower that helps one to weigh the implications of our acts to overcome our urges. The cool system helps us to find ways to draw attention away from our urges and find ways to address our desires more appropriately.

Ego Depletion

Research has shown self-control to be a finite tool. Long-term self-control training helps to strengthen this. Exercising self-control helps you to change over time. But short-term self-control is tight. Focusing more on your self-control just on a single aspect can find it impossible to maintain your self-control over future actions during the whole day.

Psychologists refer to that phenomenon as a loss of the ego. This happens when people use their willpower reservoir to complete the next task, making them unable to assemble any self-control.

6.7 Health Benefits

Self-control is also essential for sustaining healthy behaviour patterns. What you eat for meals, how often you work out, and whether you regularly go to the doctor are all decisions that are affected by your self-control levels and that have the potential to impact your quality of life.

Researchers have shown that self-control may have a variety of possible safety and wellness influences:

• In one research, adolescents with higher self-control rates were less prone to get overweight through puberty.

• Another analysis showed that people who exhausted their energy on an external activity were much more likely to cede to the reward when a treat was eventually offered.

• Studies have since found that adolescents who are dealing with self-control throughout adolescence are often more prone to consume alcohol and narcotics in high school.

Although self-control is obviously essential to sustaining healthier habits, some researchers agree that overstating the value of willpower may be dangerous.

The idea that self-control itself may help us accomplish our objectives will cause people to excuse themselves for not being able to escape temptation. This may even contribute to feelings of acquired helplessness when people believe they can't do something to alter a circumstance. As a result, people may give up in hurdles quickly or simply stop trying.

Motivation and Monitoring

Lack of motivation isn't the only factor affecting the achievement of goals. If you are working towards a goal, there need to be three major elements:

1. There has to be a clear objective and the desire to change. Having an uncertain or overbearingly general objective (losing weight) and lacking motivation can fail. With a strong purpose, you are more able to achieve a precisely specified target (losing 10 pounds).

2. You have to monitor your behaviour regarding achieving the target. It isn't enough just to set the target. Every day you need to track your actions and ensure you are achieving the tasks

you need to do to accomplish that target.

3. You need willpower. An important aspect of reaching every objective is to be able to monitor your behaviour. Fortunately, evidence shows that there are actions that individuals should take to increase their accessible willpower.

6.8 Tips for Improving Self-Control

That is an efficient way to improve the most out of your self-control available.

Avoid Temptation

Avoiding temptation makes sure you don't "use" your existing self-control before it's really needed.

If consuming, smoking, investing, or indulging in any other unhealthy behaviour, one way to escape pressure is to find a safe diversion. Go on a stroll, call a buddy, put in a bag of washing, or do whatever it takes to keep your mind off the stuff that is now enticing you.

Plan Ahead

Remember potential circumstances that could weaken your commitment. If you meet pressure, what measures would you take to stop giving in? Studies have shown that proactive

preparation will boost motivation even in circumstances where individuals have encountered ego-depleting results.

For starters, if you think you're having a hard time managing those snack attacks in the late afternoon, eat a well-balanced lunch filled with lots of fruit, calcium, and whole grains that will leave you feeling full.

Practice Using Self-Control

Although your restraint can become exhausted in a brief period, you can boost your resilience over time by consistently participating in activities that allow you to exercise self-control. Assume self-control as a muscle. Although hard labour will, in the short term, drain the muscle, the muscle can get stronger with time as you continue working on it.

The popular games "red light, green light," or "freeze dance" will help children from an early age develop self-control.

Focus on One Goal at a Time

Generally, an inefficient strategy is to set a number of targets at once (such as having a list of New Year's resolutions). Depleting one part of the willpower will decrease self-control in other regions. Choosing one particular target is better, and concentrating the attention on it. Once you switch the behaviour patterns required to achieve a goal into habits, you

won't need to put as much effort into maintaining them. Instead, you may use your money to achieve certain targets.

Meditate

Meditation is a great way to reinforce your musculature self-control. If you're fresh to meditation, a meditation on mindfulness is a perfect way to continue studying how to become more self-conscious so that you can help avoid the temptations. This technique can also help you to learn how to delay your thinking, which can help you manage any gut impulses that interfere with your self-control.

Remind Yourself of the Consequences

Just as self-control can ensure success and enhance your overall health, a lack of self-control can adversely affect your self-esteem, education, professional life, finances, relationships, and general health and well-being. Remembering the effects will help you feel focused when trying to manage your self-regulation.

A Word

Self-control is an important skill that enables us to regulate behaviour so that we can achieve our long-term objectives. Studies have also shown that self-control is not only essential

to achieving goals. Although self-control is a finite resource, work often shows there are strategies you can do to boost your willpower over time and to enhance it.

6.9 Self-Control Affirmations

My emotions and opinions are completely beyond my power.

I do maintain absolute influence over my emotions and feelings.

I now have the complete power of my feelings.

I should have strength and self-control.

I keep my relationships with myself true to religion.

I am filled with self-control, only in the most positive ways for me, with even the most desirable explanations for me to be so, now and forever, incredibly simple, utterly effortless, incredibly content! So hallelujah!

All the addictions and bad behaviours are ineffective over me. Both addictions and bad behaviours are curative. With tons of self-control, I have powerful and perfectly fine will power — all of the time, I have perfectly good health.

6.10 Exercise Affirmations

It doesn't have to be hard and painful to keep to your exercise schedule. By using these positive affirmations to overcome the usual patterns of thought that keep you from being someone who is always motivated to exercise, you could even prepare yourself to be seamlessly and instinctively encouraged to exert.

Read through to the sheet, and choose from each category a few affirmations. Take them at face value or save the list on your mobile phone, so that you can use them quickly every day. Put time aside each day when you finally wake up and read about your selected affirmations first. This will prepare your mind set and start to rewrite your patterns of thinking. Do the same before going to bed at night; this is very effective in having to send such affirmations to your sub consciousness right before you lie down.

You will completely change the way your mind thinks about exercise with consistent use by becoming somebody who is generally motivated to work hard, loves working out and living a healthy lifestyle and always tends to stick to their workout regimen.

Start today and encounter for yourself whether positive affirmations could be beneficial.

Any extra fat dissipates from the body.

All my workouts are hard and focused.

As my body has become thinner, I feel a strong deal of liberty and liveliness.

One of my top goals in my lifetime is to remain healthy and strong.

Exercising every day leaves me feeling awesome!

Exercising every day makes me feel happy and appealing.

Dancing enhances my vibrancy and liberates my conscience.

Every small decision I take pushes me to my perfect body.

I'm getting extra nimble and sinewy each day.

I get full performance every day by improving the strength of my workout sessions.

I look healthier and prettier every single day.

I optimize my physical capabilities every single day.

My body has become thinner and stiffer every single day.

My body is ever tougher and slimmer every day.

My body is getting pretty young and bigger and stronger each day.

My muscles are gaining strength and much more recognized each day.

My muscles get better and stiffer every single day.

I become fuller and healthier and happier every single second of the day.

Each exercise in which I engage helps me achieve my ideal body weight.

I develop more muscle each time I work out and lose more fat.

Exercising has as much for my body as it does for my state of mind.

Exercising enhances my positive self-image.

Exercising is the greatest relief pitcher of stress ever thought up.

Exercising helps make my body feel strong and vital.

Exercising activates endorphins, helping to make me a lot happier.

Exercising is revitalizing my body and strengthening my mind.

Exercising tones my body and build up my self-esteem.

Exercising every day brings me great strength.

Daily exercising enhances my mental state.

Exercising is enjoyable and enlivening.

Exercising is among my preferred relievers of stress.

Exercising rejuvenates; it gives me an abundance of resources.

I still take the time to work out.

I still search for ways to work out my body.

I'm always giving myself time to get better my body.

After I exercise, I every time extend out my musculature.

I'm a muscular machine that is lean, mean.

I'm adding years of health to my existence by doing daily workouts.

I'm still searching for different ways of keeping healthy and enjoyable.

I am pleased with my physical appearance and tone.

I'm extremely flexible and svelte.

I am incredibly versatile.

I'm incredibly proud of my stunning figure.

Every day I feel better and fitter.

Each day I look much lighter.

6.11 Positive affirmations for health and healthy habits

I am grateful that I stick to my healthy eating habits.

I'm associated with my body, and I appreciate maintaining it healthy.

My positive outlook is helping me stay healthy.

I'm physically, mentally, and emotionally stable, and I'm appreciative.

My lifelong priority is to be productive and healthy.

My lifestyle change is to be healthy.

My healthy living helps me feel incredibly good.

I look forward to a positive mentality and for a healthy person.

I love becoming productive, and that helps me sound wonderful.

I enjoy my life, and my healthy choices help me in achieving my desired look.

I am grateful that I have found time for self-care and healthy living.

I hope I will shift my behaviours to healthy ones.

I love to work out, as I feel amazed.

6.12 Healthy eating affirmations

I eat a healthy diet and enjoy being energy-filled.

By healthy eating, going to sleep enough, and exercising, I end up taking care of my body.

My healthful food choices enable me to relax and enjoy deep sleep.

I enjoy healthy meals because that's the only meal I'm looking for.

I'm nourishing my body with the right food I love.

I just eat a healthy diet, and my body has much more energy to show its own gratefulness.

I only want to make healthy choices and get my body nourished.

Positive statements are worthless in the absence of practice.

Using inspirational affirmations will also encourage us to hold

our target current, to reassure us that we will achieve what we desire and sustain a good outlook, but we must bear in mind that we do need to put some effort into it.

6.13 Affirmations for Confidence and Self-Esteem

For all the various aspects of your life where optimistic affirmations will make a change, trust is the main field.

As noted previously, affirmations operate by taking unpleasant emotions, such as suspicions, worries, and anxieties, and gradually transforming them into more optimistic feelings.

Everything should work out for me.

I'm winning.

The instruments that I need to be effective are in my hands.

No one gets the work done faster than me.

I trust in my leadership skills.

Some people aren't taking advantage of me.

I have faith in my credentials.

I don't worry about being wrong.

Luck is within my grasp.

I am sure that many are there.

My guiding force would be effective.

Any performance isn't going to make me jealous. My day is coming.

I'll chat with self-assurance and trust.

If I don't have the energy or the ability to move, I'll say, "Sorry."
The only human being that can kill me is me.

I fear being special.

Every wish that I have is achievable.

I'll be relaxed with my own body, even outside of my comfort zone.

When I fail, so I'm going to lose positively.

My commitment knows no bounds.

6.14 Mantras

What is the Mantra?

Mantras are terms, phrases, or acronyms that can help you concentrate and intensify meditation while also trying to unite you with greater power. Reiterating the mantras, you connect and feel the energy inside you and around you. In order to promote inner harmony, they are aligned with mysticism and meditation and work at freeing the mind from thought. Mantras will provide you with help while you need it most-warmth, encouragement, reassurance, strength, a sense of peace, or an energy burst-and they can be done everywhere, anywhere.

The words in mantras are carefully formulated to provide you with a way to be present and move through a given situation. Incorporating mantras into your everyday life can make you become more centered and concentrated, and more prepared to turn potential obstacles into opportunity gates.

Examples of mantras involve single terms like "Om," "peace," or "love," or Sanskrit phrases like "Om Namah Shivaya," which can be translated as bowing to our own highest selves.

The History of Mantras

Mantras are on the most ancient practices with the mind-body. We have been present for over 3,000 years, but in the last 150 years, we have not been completely explored. This is because a good portion of the mantras was written in Sanskrit's ancient Hindu language, and kept private to maintain their quality. Though Sanskrit is not spoken today, it

is held alive very much by mantras practice.

Sanskrit mantras were developed as a therapeutic device and spiritual development method. We have been used to heighten wealth, stability, power, defence, energy, and affection. Thousands of mantras were recorded over the course of history. Sanskrit mantras can be considered to be close to an everlasting flame. When you recite a Sanskrit mantra, you not only tap into the energy of the words but also the level of consciousness that those who repeated it before you put into words.

Today, mantras from Sanskrit grab the attention of neuroscientists and mind-body research teams. Most of them are researching the influence on the total quality of life and well-being of a positive mind, and mantras can certainly help to facilitate a positive outlook.

6.15 How Mantras Work & Its Benefits

Mantras allow you to shoulder your energy. Directing your attention to a constructive, compassionate way will help you minimize the tension that we all know has detrimental effects on our bodies. Positive thinking and self-talking, in fact, can:

- Make your life longer

- Underside Depression Rates

- Makes you calm

- Make it more immune to the common cold

- Boost both physical and psychological health

- Rising chance of death from heart failure

- Give you more ability to cope with life's obstacles

Mantras are like herbal items for strength when done daily. "Mantras help ready the energy centers (chakras) to absorb and utilize vast quantities of divine force," according to Therapeutic Mantras. Other potential advantages of reciting mantras include:

- Remove Subconscious Feelings

- Growing stillness

- You change your mind for the better

- Increased health, awareness and universal linkage

6.16 How to Use a Mantra?

While mantras are merely repeatable words or phrases, there is an art to practicing them more effectively. Here are a few suggestions for mantras being incorporated into everyday life.

Build Holy Domain

Pronounce them correctly

Practice regularly

Happily recite the mantras

Trust in Words

Integrate mantras into your everyday life

Say thanks

A few of the examples are

AUM – The ultimate motto, often known internationally as OM. With that powerful sound, every mantra begins. If chanted correctly this simple 3 letter word has a life-changing effect on you.

Lakshmi Mantra: Aum Srhim Hrim Maha Lakshmi Namaha.

This chant is devoted to Lakhsmi, Goddess of Capital.

Lakhsmi is the symbol of abundance and riches in the Indian Pantheon of Gods and Goddesses, a very powerful and meaningful one.

The GUM sound is the Bija rhythm, or the primary vibrations that assimilate Lord Ganesha's strength.

You chant this mantra, 108 times preferably, anytime you face the certain hurdle or threat in life, and you want to be effective with whatever you continue pursuing.

6.17 Why are mantras powerful?

The causes are various and logical. Let's discuss it one by one.

1. The Sanskrit is also quite vibrating.

2. Mantras are rather burdened with strong power

3. Mantras can get easily to your sub consciousness

4. Exponential rate sharpens your focus

5. Offers also other safety advantages

6. Mantras work about your body's energy scheme

1. The Sanskrit is also quite vibrating.

In brief, there's something incredible about the Sanskrit, the vibratory performance when this syntax is just great for the living thing mind and body.

The elegance of this mother tongue is how it starts to sound rhythmic and even a single sentence or audio seems so amazing as if it were a poem.

Hear easy "OM" chanting in some of the YouTube images, and

see how it looks mind-blowing. Vibrations, this is physics, can change the situation at a subatomic level.

The whole universe is moving up and down, all the cells including you, every organ throughout your body. If you know how to tune the right sound waves and energy to this whole system, you will be godlike.

Mantras are doing exactly that. Designed unique mantras to trigger particular energy centres and chakras.

Mantras get the ability to open the door inside you to an infinite sea of light, the gateway to divine energies and that renders you invincible.

2. Mantras are rather burdened with strong power

Mantras get a long tradition, stretching back to the year 1000. Most experienced people and yogis have understood different phrases of deep contemplation over the centuries.

One single slogan remained the same, untouched. Take, for instance, the Ganesha motto, that same mantra steadily declined and it has been sung for thousands of people for centuries. This makes all-powerful mantras. Right at this very moment when you're reading this message, that hundreds of people across the world are doing the same. You become a

part of the universal awareness any time you recite the refrain, you become a part of the very same power or purpose.

For this purpose Mantras are so strong

3. Mantras can get easily to your sub consciousness

Mantras make a subconscious impact on you. This is in contrast to the way affirmations work.

When you say, "I'm wealthy," you know very well that it's not true, their rational mind will strongly resist because it understands that your economic position isn't great.

But, it takes a lot of time to see any notable difference with new beliefs when re-wiring their brain. Whereas mantra functions differently. The mantra works on purpose.

For example, whenever you chant a lakshmi mantra you consciously or unconsciously ask for wealth. The purpose behind the slogan is abundance, the aim is subconsciously echoed with the slogan.

In this scenario, your conscious brain remains silent, and here you are having to take an individualized route. You don't owe the consciousness the opportunity to object, you're not explicitly claiming you're rich, just subconsciously calling for riches.

Another research is that mantra singing is a perfect way of being meditative, that's why many relate to it as meditation on mantra.

Your neural intensity goes down to a lower range due to a double-minded focus mostly on mantra. A reduced frequency spectrum indicates the brain has less active thought and a calm mind.

It just is incredibly possible to reach the subconscious as you turn off consciousness. That's why it's always advisable to chant phrases 215 times, a longer meeting of motto chanting can easily achieve a certain state of mind.

A quiet mental state has incredible benefits for the health.

4. Exponential rate sharpens your focus

Continuous singing and repeating the same mantra over and over again generate a concentration in one consciousness. Your brain is in another place and does not wander anywhere.

We don't have to remind you how critical lifetime concentration is. Vision is just like a powerful energy stream.

A concentration of one eye on everything is the main element for manifesting your wishes. Energy also helps improve your memories and maintains the brain safe.

5. Offers also other safety advantages

Chanting mantra offers unbelievable advantages. Those who recite every slogan every day would certainly have the benefits below, clearly the strength of the gain depends on how consistent you are about it.

A session of intensive OM chanting for example will give them the benefits below.

• Daily chanting helps declutter your brain

• Brings intense peace and enhanced sensitivity

• Promotes stronger secrecy and decreases distrust

• Rising brain volume, suggesting deep thinking & rehabilitation

• Standing upright and praying in Dhyana posture activates the respiratory system

• Chant tone acts like pulse treatment, contributing to the intense cure

• Deep & daily voices will adjust the expression of genes

• The left and right neurons are synchronized, meaning an extremely powerful brain

• Can even alter cell neural structure

• Turns on CSF & cleans the brain

6. Mantras work about your body's energy scheme

Have you heard of those chakras? Crown chakra is our body's energy-centres.

Such develop national centres are expected to have accumulated energy contained in them and to trigger it, every centre is correlated with a particular tone.

OM sound for example is used to trigger the chakra "Third Eye." There are seven main, and several minor, chakras. Power spreads around our skin, not only inside, but even outside of the body. Power is the bond between humanity and the world. All in this world interacts with the energy and prana at a subconscious point.

Mantras enable you to transfer the energies within us to accomplish any aim. There's a purpose behind every chant, every whenever you utter the phrase, you evoke a certain force. And then you sing, the greater the goal will be, so will the strength. That tends to help move things in the direction of the goal you want to succeed in life.

That's how magnificently Mantra operates, sound and vibration help shift the momentum.

6.18 Difference between Mantras & Affirmations

A "positive affirmation" is a word that is sometimes used synchronously with mantras, but the two have very different roots and applications. Neuroscientists created constructive affirmations in the 1970's, applying a new interpretation of psychiatry and cognitive science in order to deliberately rewire cycles of thinking towards more optimal outcomes. Affirmations may be mentioned at any point and appear to be full sentences describing what we want to obtain or be as though we actually had something at this moment.

Examples of optimistic comments involve phrases like "I am complete and fine as I am," "I burst with happiness," or "I radiate with affection."

Author Louise Hay is among the pioneers of these assertions. While mantras and affirmations have a common purpose of changing and inspiring, it is important to know what separates them from each other in order to practice mantras effectively.

Affirmations

- Drop in the 1970s,

- Psychological base

- Declaration based on the statement

- Are usually a full phrase

- Be replicated less

Mantras

- At least 3,000 years ago

- Based on Spirituality

- Declaration based on energy

- Can be as short as one syllable

- Loop more frequently in songs

6.19 Mantras and Affirmations for Each Chakra

Here are a few Chakra-specific mantras and statements you can use every day-on or off the mat throughout your procedure.

1st Chakra Vitality: Stability, Foundation, Instinct Survival

Affirmations, I am secure, and I am safe. I'm strong and sound. Life is all well.

Mantra   LAM

2nd Chakra Passion: Creativity, Sexuality and Emotions

Affirmations, I absolutely love my life. I'm imaginative and enthusiastic. I have power over my sexuality.

Mantra   VAM

3rd Chakra Purpose: Own Strength, Good Instinct, positivity

Affirmations There are no losses. I am gaining about everything that I do. I feel strong and secure. I am withdrawing judgment.

Mantra   RAM

4th Chakra Compassion: Love, Self-Acceptation, Interactions

Affirmations, I love and approve of myself genuinely. I am loving myself and letting go. I am thankful.

Mantra   YAM

5th Chakra Expression: Interaction, imagination, sincerity

Affirmations My feelings are safe to express. I'm being heard. I interact effectively and with clarification.

Mantra   HAM

6th Chakra Insight: Intuition, Intelligence, Common Thinking

Affirmations I confide in my instincts. I'm open to new ideas and new friends and novel environments. I see the big picture, and I appreciate it.

Mantra   OM

7th Chakra Connection: Cosmic Consciousness, awakening

Affirmations, I am peace, and there is harmony. The universe connects me, protects me, and supports me. I know my goal.

Mantra   OM

Chapter 07: Everything about Weight Loss

This chapter gives the detail about how you can lose weight by opting the simple and basic steps like estimating the proper serving sizes from each food group. What is the role of intermittent fasting and how it helps in reducing weight? A few of the basic steps in reducing weight are cutting down the calories, avoid consuming refined grains and cut down unhealthy fat from the diet. Other strategies to lose weight naturally are also explained in detail so that one can achieve optimum health. The methods used by most of the population which are wrong in so many ways are discussed as well in this chapter.

7.1 Estimation of Servings

Grains: 1 cup of ready-to - eat cereal, 1 slice of bread, 1/2 cup of rice or pasta cooked

Fruit: a cup of fresh fruit, 1 cup of juice of fruit or 1/2 cup of dried fruit

Vegetables: 1 cup raw or 1/2 cup cooked for serving size

Protein: 1 egg or 2 egg whites, 1/4 cup of dry beans or tofu, 1 cup of nut butter, 1/2 ounce of nuts or seeds, 1 ounce of cooked meat , poultry or fish;

Dairy (calcium-fortified goods and drinks can be replaced): serving size is 1 cup of milk or yogurt, 1.5 ounces of cheese (select low-fat or fat-free items)

Fat: 1 teaspoon of oil, 2 spoons of light salad dressing, 1 tablespoon of low-fat mayo, 1 teaspoon of soft margarine

Beverage: 6-8 (8-ounce) cups a day

7.2 Maintaining weight:

If you have gained weight, it may be tough to sustain your weight. It's indeed important to prioritize regular exercise and trying to make nutritious choices if you seek to retain your weight.

You need to insure you use as many calories as you eat to sustain your current weight. You might need to check with how much food you need to hold your current weight. Make sure you keep doing daily workout and consume lots of nutrient-dense foods.

7.3 Popular weight loss strategies

1. Cut calories

Some researchers claim that a straightforward rule helps in good weight management: If you consume less calories than you waste, you lose weight. Sounds simple, doesn't it? Why is weight loss so severe then?

• **Weight-loss over time is not a continuous occurrence.** For e.g., if you reduce calories you can lose weight for the first few weeks and then alter it. You eat the same amount of calories but you lose almost no weight at all. That's how you're losing body fluids and lean tissue as well as fat as you drop weight, your metabolism is decreasing and your body shifts in many respects. So to keep dropping weight every week you have to keep cutting calories.

• **Calories are not always calories.** For example, eating 100 calories of high fructose corn syrup can have another effect on the body unlike consuming 100 calories of broccoli. The key to successful weight reduction is to take out items that are filled with calories that don't make you feel satisfied (like candy) and replace them with foods that fill you up with nutrients rather than empty calories (like vegetables).

• **Plenty of us don't just feed enough to satisfy starvation.** We also switch to food for warmth or pain relief — which can easily ruin any weight reduction plan.

• **Cut carbs.** Another way of understanding weight reduction describes the issue as not eating so many calories but instead the way the body builds up fat after eating carbohydrates — especially the function of the insulin hormone. Starches from the diet reach the body as glucose, as you consume a meal. To maintain your blood glucose levels in check, this glucose is always burned off by your body before it consumes fat from food.

If you consume a meal that is high in carbs (for starters, tons of pasta, rice, pizza, or French fries), the body produces insulin to deal with all this glucose entering the blood stream. In addition to maintaining blood sugar rates, insulin achieves two important things: it stops the fat cells from producing fats for the body to use as energy source (because its goal is to utilize glucose) and it produces more fat cells to preserve everything that the body cannot consume. It will end in adding weight and so your body needs more calories to consume, so you eat more. Since insulin burns only carbohydrates, you savour carbohydrates, and thus a constant cycle of carbs consumption and weight gain begins. The reasoning goes that to lose weight, you have to break the pattern by reducing the carbs.

Some low-carb diets recommend combining carbohydrates with fat and protein, which may negatively impact the wellbeing over the long run. By choosing lean meats, fish and vegetarian protein sources, low-fat dairy items, and having to eat more than enough green leafy and non-starchy vegetables, you can reduce your risks if you try a low-carb diet and reduce your intake of saturated fats and Trans fats.

Cut fat

It's a staple in many foods: if you really don't like fat, don't eat it. Step down every row in the supermarket and you would be deluged by low-fat treats, meat and prepared meals. Even though our low fat choices have increased, obesity levels also have. Thus, why have low-fat diets not been successful for most of us?

1. Not all fat is harmful. In fact, healthy or "good" fats can help maintain your body, handle your emotions and combat exhaustion. Unsaturated fats contained in avocados, seeds, nuts, tofu, soy milk, and oily fish can really fill you up, and incorporating a touch of delicious olive oil to a vegetable

plate, for example, will make consuming healthier food simpler and increase the overall consistency of your diet.

2. We always make the incorrect advertising offs. All of them make the error of turning fat for hollow sugar calories and processed carbs. For example, rather than consuming whole-fat yogurt, we consume low- or no-fat versions which are filled with sugar to requite for the loss of taste. Or we switch our fatty breakfast food for a bagel or doughnut that tends to cause the blood sugar to surges quickly.

Follow the Mediterranean diet

The Mediterranean diet promotes trying to eat healthy fats and complex carbohydrates, together with significant amounts of fresh vegetables and fruits, nuts , fish, and olive oil — but only modest quantities of cheese and meat. However, the Mediterranean Diet is much more than just food. Often the main aspects are daily physical exercise and exchanging of food with the others.

Whatever weight loss tactic you attempt, staying motivated and avoiding common dieting pitfalls such as unhealthy eating is important.

7.4 The no-diet approach to weight control

You can consume healthy meals by following good dietary patterns and practicing portion management such that you receive as many calories as you need to keep your health status and well-being at your optimal weight. Weight reduction also occurs by itself naturally because you start making healthy eating decisions, such as limiting

• Food manufacturing,

• Products laden with fat,

• Pasta and white bread (replace whole grain versions instead),

• Foods with a high proportion of fat calories, such as many fast foods;

• Drinking beer.

Although nothing is completely prohibited, maintaining the portion size low and incorporating a little extra cardio to the everyday routine when you yield to the lure.

You'll be cutting down on calories by swapping those unwise eating options with healthier ones. If you introduce some regular physical activity, you have the ideal weight loss plan without having to make specific or problematic (and sometimes costly) diets. It's always important to continue consistently pursuing safe eating recommendations even though you've lost weight. This will contain adequate protein, vitamins, and minerals with minimal fat and sugar content.

7.5 How to naturally lose weight fast

Trying intermittent fasting

Several strategies supported by research can aid in weight loss, one being intermittent fasting (IF).

It is an eating pattern that requires continuous short-term fasts and meal consumption within a shorter period of time throughout the day.

Several reports have found that short-term intermittent fasting, with a period of up to 24 weeks, contributes to weight reduction in individuals who are obese.

The most popular approaches of intermittent fasting include:

• Method 16/8: Fasting for 16 hours and then eat at only an 8-hour window. The 8-hour period will be around lunch time to 8 p.m. for most individuals. A research study on this method discovered that feeding during every restricted period led to a significant fewer calories consumed by the participants and weight loss.

For non-fasting days it is possible to follow a balanced eating style to prevent over-eating.

• Diet 5:2: Fast on 2 per 7 days. Eat 500–600 calories on fasting.

• Alternative Day Fasting (ADF): Fast every day and eat regularly on non-fast days. The different version includes consuming just 25–30 per cent of the energy needs of the body on days of fasting.

7.6 Tracking your diet and exercise

When someone decides to reduce weight they will be mindful of what they consume and chug every day. A most efficient way to achieve so is to record anything they eat, either in a paper or online diet database.

Experts predicted that 3.7 billion health-app updates will be released by the end of the year in 2017. Of these the most common were diet applications, physical exercise, and weight loss. That's not beyond justification, because monitoring on-the-go improvement in physical exercise and weight reduction may be an efficient way to control weight.

One research showed that regular physical exercise monitoring has assisted with weight reduction. A review study, meanwhile, found a positive correlation between weight loss and the frequency of food intake and exercise monitoring. Also a tool that is as basic as a step counter can be a valuable weight-loss instrument.

Physical activity

Daily physical training has several advantages. This may assist with weight loss and weight stabilization; raise the Resting Energy Expenditure (REE); reinforce, expand muscles; and boost mood. Recommended in three types:

• Flexibility

• Force-training

• Aerobic exercise

Lift weights three times per week

For reducing weight with this plan, you don't need to diet so it does have additional benefits.

Through weight lifting, you'll lose loads of calories to stop slowing down your metabolism, which is a frequent side effect of weight loss.

Low carb diet tests suggest you can add a little bit of

musculature while reducing large quantities of fat mass.

Aim to go to the fitness center and lift heavy weights three or four days a week. When you're new to the workout, ask for some guidance from a Coach.

When weight training is not even a possibility for you, then you should suffice to do any aerobic exercises such as biking, walking or running, cycling, riding or surfing. Weight reduction will assist in both exercise and weightlifting.

The extent to which losing weight aided by exercise has been subject to discussion, but the benefits go well beyond burning fat. Exercise will boost your metabolism and enhance your outlook — and it's something from which you can actually gain. Go on a stroll, rest, and switch about and you'll find more time and inspiration in the weight-loss plan to handle the other moves.

Lack of decent Workout Time? Three 10-minute fitness spurts a day will be as effective as one 30-minute session.

Remember: It is better to gain something than nothing. Begin gradually, every day with minimal quantities of regular exercise. Then, you'll find it easy to be more physically involved when you start to lose weight and have more stamina.

Choose exercises you cherish. Opt to stroll with a friend, dance, hike, and ride, play Frisbee with a puppy, enjoy a basketball pickup game or play activity-based computer games with your children.

Eating mindfully

Mindful eating is a lifestyle in which people think what and where they consume food. Such exercise will offer individuals the ability to appreciate the meal they consume to sustain a healthier weight.

As most individuals experience stress, they also prefer to eat fast on the road, in the car, sitting at their offices and watching TV. As a consequence, plenty of people are scarcely conscious of the food they consume.

Mindful eating strategies entail:

• Sit down to lunch, ideally at a table: pay attention to the meal and appreciate the experience.

• Prevent disruptions while eating: do not switch on a television, a tablet or a mobile.

• Slow eating: take some time to eat and enjoy the meal. The method assists in losing weight, as it allows ample opportunity for a person's brain to understand the signs that

they have been full, and will help deter too much-eating.

• Make considered dietary decisions: select products that are full of nutrients and sustain them for hours instead of minutes.

Eating protein for breakfast

Protein can balance the hormones of hunger and make individuals feel whole. It is mainly attributed to a fall in the appetite hormone ghrelin and a spike in YY, GLP-1, and cholecystokinin satiation hormones.

Young people adult study has also found that the hormonal benefits of consuming a high-protein breakfast will continue for many hours.

Eggs, sardines, nut and seed butters, oats, quinoa porridge, and chia seed dessert are also healthy options for a high-protein meal.

Cutting back on sugar and refined carbohydrates

Swapping high-sugar foods to fruits and nuts will help.

The Western diet is disproportionately rich in refined sugar, and this has clear ties to obesity, even though the sugar is found in drinks rather than foods.

Processed carbs are products that are highly refined and no longer sustain fiber as well as other vitamins and minerals. Those involve white rice, noodles, and pizza.

Such products are easy to digest, so they rapidly turn to glucose.

Excess glucose reaches the blood and triggers the insulin release, which facilitates the accumulation of fat in the abdominal fat. This assists in gaining weight.

People will substitute refined and sugary products for healthy alternatives, whenever necessary. There are successful food exchanges which include:

• Instead of the white varieties, whole grain beans, bread and pasta

• Instead of a high-sugar snack, fruit, nuts and seed

• Herbal teas and coffee flavored with fruit, rather than high-sugar soft drinks

• Milk or milk smoothies, instead of fruit juice

Eating plenty of fiber

Dietary fiber identifies plant-based carbs unlike sugar and starch, which cannot be absorbed in the small intestines. Having lots of dietary fiber will improve the sense of fullness, which may help in losing weight.

Foods abundant in fiber include:

- Whole grown cereals, whole wheat noodles, whole grain bread, oats, rice, and rye

- Vegetables and fruits

- Pulses, peas, beans

- Seeds and nuts

Balancing gut bacteria

One emerging research area focuses on bacteria's role in weight control in the gut.

A large number and diversity of microbes, including about 37 trillion bacteria, are found in the human body.

A growing person has various varieties in their gut and different quantities of bacteria. Some styles will raise the amount of energy the individual harvests from food, contributing to weight gain and fat deposition.

Many foods may raise the amount of healthy intestinal bacteria including:

- **A large range of plants:** Growing the amount of fruits, vegetables and grains in the food can contribute to improved

fiber intake and a more balanced collection of intestinal bacteria. Consumers will strive to make sure veggies and other plant-based products make up 75% of their meal.

• **Fermented foods:** improve the role of healthy bacteria whilst preventing harmful bacteria from developing. Sauerkraut, miso, kimchi, kefir, yogurt, tempeh, and miso all comprise considerable levels of probiotics which contribute to the growth of healthy bacteria. Researchers have investigated kimchi thoroughly, and results from the research indicate it has an anti-obesity impact. Similarly, trials have shown that kefir can aid promote weight reduction in people who are overweight.

• **Prebiotic foods:** It encourages the development and function of some of the healthy bacteria that help regulate weight. In several fruits and vegetables, prebiotic fiber occurs particularly in chicory root, artichoke, asparagus, onion, leeks, garlic, banana, and avocado. It's even in cereals, including oats and barley.

Getting a good night's sleep

Numerous researches have found that it is correlated with an elevated prevalence of obesity to sleep fewer than 5–6 hours a night. There are multiple explanations for this.

Research suggests that insufficient or poor sleep tends to slow down the system wherein the body turns calories, into energy called metabolism, when metabolism becomes less efficient, the body can store energy that is wasted as fat. Furthermore, sleep deprivation can increase insulin and cortisol production which also encourages fat accumulation.

How long one sleeps often influences the production of leptin and ghrelin, the appetite-control hormones. Leptin gives messages to the brain about fullness.

7.7 Managing your stress levels

Outdoor sports can help ease stress.

Stress activates the production of hormones such as adrenaline and cortisol which at first reduce hunger as part of the body's emergency response.

If people are under intense tension, though, cortisol will linger longer in the body, which can raise their hunger and eventually cause them to consume more.

Cortisol suggests the need to refill the food reserves of the body from the natural fuel supply which is carbohydrate.

Insulin then carries glucose sugar from the blood into the

muscles and brain. Unless the individual will not use this sugar in battle or flight, the body may store it as fat.

Researchers observed that the introduction of an 8-week stress-management training plan culminated in a substantial reduction in children who are overweight and teenagers in the body mass index (BMI).

Several stress-management approaches include:

• Yoga, tai chi or mediation

• Respiratory and rehabilitation methods

• Spend some time outdoors, such as walking or growing vegetables

Control emotional eating

We're not just feeding solely to relieve appetite. Far too much, when we are depressed or nervous, we switch to food which can ruin every diet and pile on the pounds. Can you eat while you are nervous, tired or lonely? Will you eat at the end of a long day, in front of the Screen? Recognizing your emotional eating causes will make your weight-loss attempts all the better. When you feed at every point you are:

Stressed-seeking safe ways to cool down. Practice meditation, reflection or a hot water bath.

Low on energy-try some pick-me-ups mid-afternoon. Opt to stroll around the street, listen to soothing songs, or take a brief nap.

Lonely or depressed – reach out to anyone, rather than heading towards the freezer. Call a buddy that makes you chuckle, bring your dog for a stroll, or head to the store, library, or garden — where there are crowds around.

Stay motivated

Lasting weight loss includes healthy lifestyle choices and eating habits. Staying motivated:

Check for a cheering region. Social help means a lot. Programs such as weight control use group support for impacting weight loss and healthy eating for a lifetime. To have the motivation you need, seek assistance — whether in the form of a family, friends, or a counselling service.

Losing weight so quickly will lead to fatigue, drained and tired, taking a toll on your body and mind. The target for reducing one to two pounds a week though you lose fat instead of water and muscular weight.

Create targets to keep motivated. Short-term aspirations, such as fitting into a summer bikini, typically don't work as well as trying to feel more comfortable or becoming better for the sake of your family. Reflect on the rewards you'll receive by staying safe as opportunity hits.

To chart the progress using the software. Smartphone apps, fitness trackers or just keeping a newspaper can easily keep track of the food that you eat, the number of calories you eat and the weight you end up losing. Seeing the monochrome results will help you remain inspired.

Get lots of good night sleep. Sleeplessness increases the appetite such that you crave more food than regular; at the very same time, it keeps you from feeling full, causing you to want to consume more. Sleep deficiency will also have an effect on your productivity, so strive for 8 hours of consistent sleeping hours.

Take charge of your food environment

Put yourself in a position for weight-loss results by taking accountability for your eating setting: what you consume, how much you consume, and what readily accessible products you produce.

Serve small chunks accordingly. To make the servings look bigger, using tiny pots, containers, and cups. Do not eat directly from large bowls or food containers which makes it very difficult to determine how much you have consumed.

Cook your own homemade meals. It helps you to monitor both the size of the portion and what is getting into the meal. In general, restaurants and packaged foods contain much more artificial sweeteners, undesirable fat, and calories unlike home-cooked foods — plus the food portions tend to be larger.

Fast for 14 hours a day. Try eating dinner sooner in the day, and then fast till the next morning meal. Eating right while you're most busy and taking a lengthy break from your metabolism will help in weight reduction.

Eating early. Studies suggest you could even assist drop more pounds by consuming even more your total calories at morning meal, and lesser at dinner. You will improve your metabolic rate by consuming a bigger, healthier breakfast, avoid getting hungry throughout the day, and allow you further time to work up calories.

Prep the snacks and meals in advance. You can make a small portion of your own snack foods in plastic containers or bags. Eating as per plan will help you stop consuming when you're not very hungry.

Sip more of that water. Thirst can also be mistaken with appetite, and you can prevent extra calories while consuming tea.

Restrict the quantity of food you have at residence which is enticing. If you start sharing a kitchen with non-dieters, retain off sight extravagant food products.

7.8 Plateaus

Even if you eat well and do exercise, you may achieve a plateau at which your weight remains the same. Plateaus are mainly attributable to reduced energy resting (REE) expenses. Your REE tends to reduce because you eat less calories, so your body's natural requirement of energy reduces. Continue to exercise and eat well enough to support you get through time intervals without any weight reduction. Sometimes even a plateau is a way for the body to tell you may not even have to lose weight. Losing weight is not homogeneous, and its biological results are complex. If you experience emotional or physical suffering due to efforts to lose weight, express out this to friends, family or maybe a healthcare professional.

7.9 Less safe methods of weight loss:

Seek advice with a healthcare professional or registered dietitian prior to actually starting a new eating plan.

Low-calorie diets: Reducing your daily calories by less than 1400 calories per day would be detrimental, because your body adapts to a semi-hungry state and is looking for alternative energy sources. Your body eventually burns muscle tissue, in addition to fat burning. But since your heart is a muscle it will be seriously damaged by times of starvation and tamper with its regular beats. Low-calorie foods do not satisfy the dietary requirements of the body and the body can't function properly lacking nutrition.

Appetite suppressant medicines and other diet pills: "Wonder" items that irreversibly promote weight loss don't really prevail. Goods which guarantee instant or unobtrusive loss of weight would not work long term. Satiety suppressants, that often contain a psychoactive drug such as caffeine, are associated with health risks such as morning sickness, nasal dryness, agitation, anxiety, lightheaded, sleeplessness and higher blood pressure pres.

Fad diets: Most fad diets promote consuming a lot of one form of food instead of a range of foods, which may be very

harmful. Such forms of diets are also designed to manipulate consumers into wasting more on unhealthy and even unproven goods. The best approach to consume requires balanced meals, so you can receive all the nutrition the body needs for.

Liquid diets: liquid dietary products or shakes that contain fewer than 1000 calories a day could be used under very strict professional monitoring. Such foods may be unhealthy and are not nutrient effective due to excessive amounts of sugar. There is also a very poor fibre content that induces blood sugar spike and drops. Moreover, liquid diets do not reduce appetite, leading on the over-consumption of certain foods.

7.10 What's the best diet approach for healthy weight loss?

Pick up every diet book and it would falsely claim to contain all the keys to easily shed all the pounds you would like — and keep it all off. Many say that the trick is to consume less and workout more, some that fat free is the only way to get there, and some recommend leaving out carbohydrates.

The irony is that there is no "one size fits all" approach for successful safe weight reduction. What works with one

individual does not work for another because our bodies adapt differently to specific diets, based on biology and other health considerations. It is possible that choosing the best weight loss strategy for you would take time and include persistence, determination, and also some exploration with multiple diets.

Although some people react well to calorie counting or similar restrictive techniques, others react favorably to getting more liberty in organizing their weight-loss strategies. Simply avoiding fried foods or cutting back on processed carbohydrates could even set them up to succeed. So, don't be too downhearted if a regimen that worked for someone else doesn't work for you.

Remember: although there's no obvious answer to lose weight, there are still plenty of measures that can be taken to establish a healthful attitude towards food, reduce binge eating emotional triggers and sustain a healthy weight.

7.11 Keeping the Weight Off

You might have noticed the commonly cited figures that 95 percent of people trying to lose weight on a diet can recover it within a matter of years — or even months. Although there are not any concrete data to confirm this argument, it's clear that many weight-loss programs struggle in the long term. Maybe it's probably because overly stringent diets are really challenging to manage over time.

The (NWCR) National Weight Control Registry in the United States, since it was founded in 1994, has monitored over 10,000 people that have gained considerable quantities of weight and held it off over lengthy periods of time. The research showed that participants who have been effective in retaining their weight loss follow similar approaches.

• **Stay fit and active.** Prosperous dieters in the NWCR study exercise typically going to walk for around 60 min.

• **Keep a food log.** Recording your daily intake helps to keep you responsible and driven.

• **Consume breakfast every day.** It's most often cereal and fruit in the research. Consuming breakfast increases the appetite warding off craving later that same day.

• **Have more fiber than the standard** American diet, and less fat.

• **Check your scale regularly.** Trying to weigh yourself weekly may help you spot any slight weight gains, allowing

you to take appropriate corrective actions even before a problem occurs.

• **Watch less TV.** Minimizing the hours spent seated in front of the television will be a vital aspect of having a healthier lifestyle and weight gain avoidance.

7.12 Hindrances in weight loss

Relying Too Much on Water

Drinking water is fantastic for the body. Although it is also claimed that consuming additional water then you'll need to ward off thirst is a magical weight losing trick — specifically consuming 6 to 8 glasses every day or more. Nevertheless, there is little confirmation that this will be effective. This turned out that drinking water, whether warm or room temperature, just expends a small amount of calories. So focusing on this plan will not get you far from shedding pounds. On the other hand, people occasionally eat when they are really thirsty. And it is not a poor thing to quench the thirst before having a bite. It's always effective to approach for a drink of water than just a sugary drink, Pepsi or spice latte — any calorie drink can influence your quality of life, so there's no reason to think about it with water.

Sleeping Too Little — or Too Much

People put on some weight occasionally, for unexpected causes. One in four Americans isn't having enough time. And it could be that the shortage of sleep contributes to the obesity problem. Dozens of scientific studies have explored a link between obesity and sleep in infancy and several have identified a linkage. It is not clear if obesity makes it more difficult to have enough sleep or sleep which induces obesity. Many reports also aimed at people who are overweight. Such findings also indicate a correlation between increasing weight and getting more than 9 hours of sleep or below five hours. This could be due to the hormone levels. Sleep cycles influence hormones linked to hunger and energy intake-burning-leptin and ghrelin. Besides that, individuals who sleep less generally feel fatigued and far less able to do workouts. Whatever the cause might be, if you have difficulty losing weight you might like to focus on sleep quality.

Relying on Restaurant Meals

Whether you have a full life or simply aren't a lover of home cooking, you place your body at the hands of the restaurants you buy from. Also dishes marketed as "sweet" can contain more calories than you've been shopping for so several restaurants, especially smaller ones, don't mention their nutritional statistics so you can see what you're really consuming. There's even evidence that people who eat restaurant lunches outweigh those who prepare lunch at home by an average of five pounds.

Too Many Tiny Meals

You might have got to hear that trying to eat lots of small meal options all day long helps keep you fuller for longer without any excess calories. Yet to confirm this, there is barely any statistical evidence. Not only are tiny, daily meals stressful for preparing, but they may potentially end up backfiring, forcing you to consume more and then once you start feeding, it may be hard to quit. If that is how you want to fuel your body, go for it. But it doesn't matter if your restricted-calorie diet is ingested all day long, or just three or four times a day. The most crucial part is having to eat a healthy diet with the proper calorie count.

Taking a Seat — All Day Long

Will that sound familiar to you? You are riding in the car to work, and going to a workplace where you are working for much of the day. You're worn out when you get home, and just want to — can you guess? Only sit down, maybe watch some television. All that sitting means your body doesn't move as much as it should for the best outcomes for your health. Studies have shown that those who spend more time sitting are more likely to weigh. But some studies say weighing more will lead people to sit more frequently. It's a complex process that affects the other, but here's something that's well known: while you're seated, you're not driving, doing housework or standing up and running around a ton. All this energy that should be used eating up a few more calories by exercise, just through having a rest, health is sapped. And it can only benefit to take out more room each day to pass.

Overdoing Alcohol

Alcoholic beverages can expand your middle section more than you know. A beer, or two a day is popular among many Americans. But it sure does add up. Anyone that consumes two shots of vodka a day per week contributes about 1,400 calories to their diet — that's most calories in a day! And add still more wine and beer. Two bottles of wine a week contribute about 1,600 calories to the weekly count, and about 2,100 beers a day. So if you're willing to get serious about weight loss consider putting down the mug of beer for a while.

Rewarding Exercise with Food

Some people think that they can justify the extra help of pasta at dinner by working out. That may not however be the case. When we work out, we tend to overestimate the calories that we burn and technology doesn't help. Researchers find in one analysis that the typical aerobic unit overestimates on typical calories burnt by 19 per cent. In that research, elliptical machines were the worst offenders, an average of 42 per cent overestimating. That adds up to over a year's work out! Fitness bands have shown identical issues.

Not Planning for Mealtime

To every busy person, grab-and-go meals are enticing and most of us suits the description. It's all too easy to overeat high-calorie convenience food when your family and job take all your time and attention. What's worse is that, fast food is low in fiber and fiber is the key nutrient that keeps you full longer, meaning you'll just want to add an extra cheeseburger or soda to that order to feel satisfied. The approach is ahead thought. Start by preparing your own convenience foods ahead of time. Look for high-fiber, easy-to-prepare alternatives such as beans and salads which can be whipped up as soon as hunger hits. As you get better at this, you'll start seeing your waistline shrink, as well as the cost of your food.

Turning to Snacks When You're Stressed Out

Have you ever learned of emotional eating? Eating can become an effort to fill an emotional vacancy within your life when you're stressed out. Sometimes this includes excessive snacking on high-calorie products, piling on pounds. One study had hair locks investigated for the cortisol stress hormone. For candidates who showed signs of long-term stress, they found a significant relationship between the waist size and high body-mass index (BMI). None of this has a bright side to it. You can ease stress without having your wardrobe stretched out. Exercising can be the best way to both burn stress and lose weight. And relaxing techniques such as meditation, yoga, deep breathing and massage can bring peace to your life — no calories needed.

Thyroid Problems

Weight gain is often linked to an underlying health condition known as hypothyroidism. Hypothyroidism comes in when very little thyroid hormone is released by the thyroid gland. It's more growing amongst women. Hypothyroidism symptoms may be subtle and may include a slow heart rate, thinning hair, a puffy face, a heavy voice, exhaustion, depression, muscle pain, and feeling cold when other people don't. The positive thing for those struggling with this disease is that regular medicine is treatable. And if those things sound similar and you would like to be checked out, speak with the doctor about the matter. A physician will help you test your thyroid hormone levels and prescribe a prescription or a doctor.

Baby on the Way

Once they are pregnant women do and can put on weight. It is estimated that a fit, the pregnant lady would gain around 25 to 35 lbs. Whether you are obese or overweight, then those statistics will be smaller. When you are seeking more than that and consider yourself achieving more, there are many strategies to hold your body in control. Aim to take a stroll between meals. Eat healthy, natural foods such as lean proteins, natural grains, fruits and vegetables, which are perfect for you as well as your new-born-to-be. There are also lots of workouts that are safe for pregnant moms, but there are those that can be prohibited, please speak to the practitioner about it before starting a new program.

Menopause and Weight Gain

Menopause and the physiological shifts that it entails in several respects depend on women's bodies. And, indeed, there is always one additional is body fat. Menopause results in slowing the metabolic rate, meaning that women gain an average extra 10 pounds during this time span. Menopause also influences the way the body allocates its fat, which is of concern. Throughout that time, fat is much more likely to be retained across the belly, and that has implications for heart health and therefore can trigger insulin issues. Will menopause imply you're condemned to being fat? Neither at all. Even, food and exercise will help you shed weight. One research tracked 17,000 post - menopausal people and placed them on a diet full of fruits, vegetables and whole grains. Three times more often the ones on the diet will lose weight. What's more, the hot flashes were also less severe. Other studies observed more than 500 premenopausal females who had their calories decreased by around half with which their physical condition improved. On average some women had narrower waists and after five years were more prone to be at or under their initial weight.

Prescription Drugs Can Cause Weight Gain

Prescribed medications often interact with other facets of your well-being, like this one. Steroids can get in the path of weight reduction as they can mess with your appetite and leave you feeling hungry. Antihistamines are a particular culprit. They help your hunger to intensify. Although certain antihistamines might be more effective for this than others, there have been no trials providing side-by - side associations among antihistamines and appetite, and whether you want to stop hunger and hold the hay fever at bay, you'll need to submit experimentation before such tests are being conducted.

Relying on Weight Lifting

There's really nothing inaccurate with using vigorous exercise to sculpt your body or build muscle. But if you focus on weightlifting for your weight loss plan, you may be disheartened. There are two types of exercise here anyway basically. One is aerobic, and includes activities aimed at getting your heart pumping over even a prolonged period of time, such as cycling, jogging, and rowing, walking or running and hopping rope. The other is anaerobic, where you work out for a brief period at a high intensity, making your heart beat much more fiercely. Such exercises help the body work best in short bursts, with weightlifting included. Researches appear to show aerobic workouts are the clear champion for losing fat. For a longer duration, they maintain your heart rate going, which contributes to much more burned energy, and it is equivalent to weight loss. The anaerobic activity also benefits but just not quite that much. So while you are good at both exercises, they serve multiple functions.

And if you're focusing both-in on weightlifting, the fat-burning potential of aerobic exercise is leaving out.

Falling for Fake Health Food

Often the fast food barely qualifies as a nutritious product. Just how infuriating! Through finding such health-food fakers you will spare yourself the annoyance.

• Juices and smoothies: it's produced from vegetables and fruits that don't keep it good. These apparently healthier options take on one of the greatest benefits of fruit and veggies — fibre — and remove it, most of the time leaving large amounts of sugar behind. Green juices are possibly good choices if you need your remedy. Smoothies can also include ice cream, or high-fat dairy, but closely review the list of ingredients.

• Power Bars and cereal bars: Well, when you see something like this on the local supermarket shelf, you only think about runners and long walks. Yet there is as much sugar in the normal power or cereal bar as in a chocolate product.

• Multi-Grain and Wheat Breads: This bread is found on the store aisle and you barely know all concerning whole grain. Wheat is a grain, after all, right? The concern is that these are not nutritious whole grain bread until explicitly specified by the label. When in question, search for fibre content on the nutrition data. Whole grain bread should really have around 3-5 grams per slice of fibre which makes it a nutritious option. Sometimes these health-food fakers have 1 gram or lower.

Drinking Empty Calories

Don't drink calories either! Chugging a carbonated drink, juices, energy drink, chocolate milkshake, or sport beverages every now and then during the day is quick to get into the addiction. If you are consuming the calorie-free type, each provides calories. Yet on two different ends losing weight is tougher. The first concern refers to food. Although sweet beverages contribute calorie intake to your regular count, they don't help satisfy the appetite. The body scarcely recognizes them as food, and you can quickly drink many without having to feel full. The other thing is that only a few sugar-sweetened beverages a day easily add up. Data reveals 1 in 4 Americans consume at least 200 calories a day. If you add it to your daily intake over the duration of a year, that's 73,000 calories. That is more than 20 pounds of body fat equivalent to that. And even cutting those beverages out of your diet will help you shed a huge amount of weight in a year.

Not Asking for Help

Losing weight and holding that off can be a daunting struggle because if you don't seek out for support, the chances are very much against you. Luckily there are several highly skilled professionals conditioned to help you get to your healthy body weight and stay there in the particular ways you have to. Your healthcare provider is the first one to go in. Your doctor can give prescriptions depending on your experience and personal healthcare needs. A doctor may refer you to a fitness instructor, who is responsible for designing workout routines customized to your body and capacity. A psychiatrist can assist by identifying the environments that contribute to stress eating as well as other harmful lifestyle habits of your life. Dietitians will offer encouragement and suggestions on meal preparation, and also accompany you shopping to find the perfect items that will not impede your trip but help. Finally, reducing stress with the assistance of a meditation or yoga teacher could have a strong effect on your current health if you are one of the many people engaged in stress eating.

Dining in front of the TV

While it doesn't load on pounds all on its own, more and more time you put munching in front of the TV, the more certainly you 're going to eat without a consciousness. That's dangerous for someone who tries to shed weight without modifying their eating patterns. Studies have shown that eating distracted tends to mean having to eat extra. You seem to neglect what you did as well as how much you consumed while you're tired so that ensures you 're more prone to binge later on. Having to tell your brain when you are satisfied requires approximately 20 minutes for the stomach so calming down and cherishing food makes you remain satisfied with lesser. And consider feeding without interruption, instead of munching in front of the Screen. Take short bites, and chew well. Set a 20-minute timer before going back for second utilization. Another technique is feeding with your less-dominant side, which encourages you to watch out.

Failing to Set Goals

If it's making money, strengthening your marriages, or losing weight, resolutions will aid if you want to improve something in life. Setting targets may help you shed your extra weight, but retaining your healthy, safer lifestyle may be much more critical. But there are a couple of regulations that can be useful when establishing those goals. Firstly, make your targets specific. It's not sufficient just to intend to consume little — decide how less, particularly. What things do you cut off from your diet? What is it you are going to add? How frequently?

Still, if your objective is quantifiable, you'll have a specification to use in deciding whether or not you've been true to your target. Ultimately, make sure that your target is worthy of tracking — something like dropping a certain amount of pounds over time. If you don't reach any of your objectives, so another crucial step is to accept yourself and continue over again. Each day provides a fresh chance to continue making the change you desire and your body requires in terms of wellness.

Chapter 08: Myths, Facts and Mind Exercises

This chapter consists of all the myths and facts related to weight loss in detail. These are the myths that are taken as facts, which ultimately mislead the person trying to lose weight. So these are discussed in depth in this chapter. Strategies to reduce the appetite, in the long run, are also mentioned so that it would be helpful for a person to attain the goal and retain it. Also, the mind exercises are mentioned to practice so that you can train your mind accordingly.

8.1 Myths and Facts about Diet

Weight reduction Implies Fat Loss.

If you see a dramatic drop on the scale, particularly overnight, then you can be excited to lose weight so fast. Although this doesn't automatically mean it's fat loss — it may be water weight. "[Water weight] is excess water that falls inside the cells throughout the tissues, joints, and bodily fluids. It's a different weight than body fat; it's not relevant to absorb or spent calories. An increase in body weight may be contributing to consuming so much salt or a shift in hormones, which may be reduced easily by exercising without drinking enough fluid (which seems somewhat intuitive, but it's true!).

Breakfast is a must to lose weight.

Studies suggest that skippers appear to gain much more than eaters for breakfasts. That's presumable because people consuming breakfast are much more inclined to have certain good lifestyle behaviours, though. In reality, a 4-month study examined breakfast habits among 309 adults and found no impact on weight if the respondents ate or missed breakfast. It's also a misconception that eating breakfast can improve metabolism, and that consuming several tiny meals can help you consume more calories every day. Eating when you're hungry is best, and stopping when you're full. Eat breakfast if you like, but don't expect it to have a major impact on your weight. Although it is possible that breakfast skippers appear to weight much more than breakfast eaters, regulated trials indicate that weight loss does not really affect whether you consume or miss breakfast.

A regime of radical exercise seems to be the only way of losing weight

Not quite so. Effective weight management means making minor changes to which you will commit for a long period.

That means being more productive in your regular activities, physically. Adults could get at least 150 minutes of physical exercise a week, such as a brisk walk or running, though for those that are overweight would definitely require more to reduce weight than that.

You'll need to utilize more calories than you ingest to reduce weight. This can be accomplished by choosing to eat less, moving more, or, at best, combining both.

Only reducing carbs is the key to reducing weight.

If you're looking to consume a balanced diet, you can't abandon carbohydrates. The 2015 American Dietary Guidelines suggest three dietary patterns: the traditional American approach, the traditional Mediterranean approach, and the balanced vegetarian approach.

"One of these balanced eating practices is focused on carbohydrate-rich ingredients, such as veggies (which include beans and lentils), fruits, and whole grains. So note the fiber is carbohydrate. Your fiber consumption will plunge if you skip carbohydrates.

Snacking is always a negative thing.

The positive thing is that you will not have to suffer through weight loss. "The belief you're not allowed to consume during meals is a fallacy. You probably have heard that little tone in your mind telling you not to disrupt your desire to eat once your stomach starts groaning. But getting snacks between meals can potentially make you eat less and stay away from the temptation to eventually over-eat or binge. In fact, dietitians often suggest getting five smaller meals a day, rather than eating all of your calorie intake in one seat.

Several of the major reasons why snacking does have a bad reputation is because of decisions we make from, say, a vending machine packed with chips, cookies, candy bars, and other delightful treats — and fattening —. The positive thing is that we don't just chomp on chocolate bars after 4 p.m.

When you like to plunge into a packet of crisps once you're starving, consider healthier snacks instead — think, for instance, of small quantities of fruits, veggies, and beans — and aim to consume items you usually don't have at mealtime.

People ought to show the will to reduce weight.

A person's progress or inability to lose weight is not a measure of their reservoir of willpower. There are several variables that play into a person's size — genomics, climate, and otherwise — and an increasing proof of evidence suggests that as individuals lose weight, biological aspects come into play, making things difficult for them to hold the weight off when it's gone.

When an individual loses a large amount of weight, their digestion becomes out of proportion, and their hunger rises proportionally, allowing them to consume around 100 more calories per every two pounds lost. Although this doesn't mean that holding weight off over the long term is difficult, it does imply that trying to do that is by no way a result of the determination, dedication, or hard work.

Healthier products cost more.

Healthier foods may seem costlier than their unhealthy alternative solutions. And, because you're looking to swap foods with safer options, you'll definitely notice that the recipes would cost less. Selecting cheap meat cuts and combining them with cheaper substitutes such as rice, peas, and frozen veg, for example, would help it go faster in casseroles or stir-fries.

You'll have progress right away.

You did all the right things to shed pounds: you eliminated junk food, loaded on nutritious eating and lean protein, and perused Eat This, Not That! For diet ideas and quick trades. You haven't even seen the scale budge yet, though. This is because everyone is distinctive from each other. While some people want to reduce weight reduction down to a "calories in, calories out" method, the fact is that the human body is far more complex than that. An individual has a specific metabolism, collection of hormones, environmental influences, and possible underlying health problems that may all play a role in how frequently he or she loses weight. Therefore, it may take time to see measurable effects. That doesn't mean it won't happen; while having to wait for the measurement to move, you just have to be consistent and patient. The second you continue to eat good, don't assume to see immediate weight reduction impact.

You could target areas of trouble.

You might be very anxious about the fat on your buttocks, and want to trim them down as soon as possible. We have the unfortunate news: that's not feasible. You might lose weight eventually, of course, by consuming the best meals and doing enough activity, but there's no hint about when the fat would be shed. Each body is special, and the targeting of fat loss from particular body areas via diet is unlikely. With that said, workouts can tone muscular strength, which may translate to slimmer-looking specific areas of the body.

Eating through the night makes you gain weight.

Put the myth of the diet to rest. There's no conclusive evidence that late-night meals result in weight gain. We realize that so many calories are triggering weight gain, and often night eaters prefer to over-eat and select high-calorie products. Consuming close to bedtime can still cause stomach upset and digestive problems. So prefer to adhere to regular mealtimes — and earlier —

Coffee isn't right for you.

That is a food myth that has only been demolished. Coffee is a secured part of a balanced diet when taken properly (2 to 3 cups per day), and adds antioxidant phytochemicals. Indeed, research suggests that coffee can help lower the risk of diabetes, gallstones, Parkinson's disease, including some types of cancer. Nonetheless, maintain coffee calories in order. Stay away from milk, sugar, and syrup-flavored drippings.

Certain sweets are worse than the others.

Table sugar, agave, honey, and high fructose corn syrup add calories (approximately 48 and 64 per tbsp). Investigation shows so far that our bodies simultaneously consume processed sugars such as high-fructose corn syrup and table sugar. Instead of eliminating one specific form of sugar, aim to restrict all sorts of artificial sugars, such as those in soft drinks, sweets as well as other desserts.

Shift to sea salt for sodium reduction

Think that converting to sea salt would conserve sodium? Sorry, this, too is, a dietary myth. Fine dining salts by weight have almost the same sodium as the regular simple table salt. Instead, add some spice with chili pepper, herbs, and spices. In fact, we obtain about 75% of our daily salt consumption from packaged and dried products (not the salt shaker) such as soups, seasonings, sauces, cheeses, and tinned food.

To chip off pounds, drink more water.

There's really no wonder that water is essential to your body — but an aid to losing weight? Not quite. If drinking water helps keep you away from high-calorie beverages, it can help you lose weight, of course. But introducing additional water to your intake, without doing anything else, doesn't make much difference in reducing the scale amounts.

The less you eat fat, the better.

For the body to survive, it requires three nutrients: protein, carbohydrates, and fats. Better for you, fats contained in foods such as nuts, beans, seafood, avocado, olives, and low-fat dairy give you strength, help regenerate cells, and generate the hormones required. Saturated and trans fats are the fats to constrain or prevent, found in foods such as butter, high-fat dairy, red meat, and many refined foods.

Prevent refined grains

We know that whole grains are perfect for us because fibre, vitamins, minerals, and phytochemicals are loaded in them. That just doesn't mean that you have to dissect all the packaged grains. At times, such as when the body recovers from a gastrointestinal infection, it can take processed grains. And the folic acid fortification in certain processed grains. While whole grains are the healthiest choice, you can also give allowance for some packaged fortified grains.

Athletes need a lot of protein.

Everybody knows an athlete needs loads and loads of protein to develop muscle and strength, right? Well, probably not. Most American diets also supply athletes with plenty of protein. The real secret to enhancing athletic resilience and muscle is getting enough calories, focusing on intensive training, and getting a snack that contains carb and protein (such as non-fat chocolate milk) shortly after such an intense muscle workout. Need not to apply specific powders, bars,

and fortified foods!

Sugar can trigger children to be hyperactive.

That myth is so common that it would seem incredibly difficult not to be true. But most evidence indicates that glucose doesn't get hyperactive all babies. So why it is that children jump off the walls at kids' parties? This is not the dessert; it is actually the thrilling surroundings. Even, keep an eye on how much sugars the children consume. Too many treats leave no space for healthy eating.

Carbs result in gaining weight.

Quit believing the myth of that diet. Not that all carbs to you are harmful. Yet it seems people are gaining pounds on low-carbohydrate diets, right? These diets also restrict calories nearly always, so fewer calories stack up to fewer pounds over time irrespective of how much of the calories are from fat, protein, or carbs.

Too much sugar can lead to diabetes.

Worried your passion for cake or candy would contribute to diabetes? Avoid thinking about food theory. If you have no diabetes, drinking sugar isn't going to lead you to have the disorder. However, what does increase your risk of diabetes is being inactive and overweight. So do yourself a favor: cut

back on the calories that are empty, sugar, and move.

8.2 Tips for identifying food misinformation

• First, if it seems too amazing to be real, and it is almost certainly true.

• Second, consider asking yourself, "who's saying that?" Is that person biased in making the statement? Are they attempting to market a specific product? Was this knowledge based on a little limited research?

• The significant weight loss or routine maintenance is not a secret ingredient. We have known that eating healthy perfectly right and particularly exercising matters.

8.3 Factors lowering the appetite in long-term

Stress

It's difficult to overlook old fashioned stress eating whenever it comes to variables that impact eating. But different kinds of stress can affect different people in different ways.

Major stressors — such as war, famine, and traumatic injury — are linked with an increased incidence of cultivating psychological problems, such as severe depression and stress disorder, which are both linked to alterations in the desire to eat, which explored the biological cause for feeding and eating disorders.

But it's less clear whether the information on slight stimuli — the kind's individuals face on a daily basis — can activate hunger. Around 40 percent of people acknowledge eating is a result of stress in polls, but another 40 percent claim they feel a decline in their appetite as a result of stress. As for the 20 percent remaining? They do not mention any impact.

It's still uncertain what tends to trigger stress-induced feeding inside the body. Historically, cortisol [stress hormone] has been primarily linked to stress-induced eating. However, this connection has been backed up by research demonstrating that higher levels of cortisol — resulting in either medicines or disease — could impact metabolism. Mild stress also shows a significant rise in cortisol levels, but these rises are much narrower and do not last as long, so it is not completely clear how much cortisol has increased.

Somewhat, "ghrelin, and possibly leptin, in response to chronic stress also likely bring about changes in calorie consumption and weight. The best statistics for that, however, are in rodents, not in human beings.

Mindfulness-based strategies are likely the strongest research for individuals who would like to decrease stress eating. The proof in this field is not conclusive, though. Mindfulness "is that when a person attempts from time to time to be conscious of whatever he or she experiences emotionally and psychologically. However, in relation to being attentive, maintaining a record about what you consume is another method that will help you track how food consumption responds to shifts in emotions.

Sleep

A number of studies have found that not having enough sleep raises appetite; for example, sleep deprivation will contribute to ghrelin increase and leptin reduction.

Shifts in the leptin and ghrelin thresholds are assumed to be more involved in homeostatic hunger, although there is growing evidence that hedonic hunger may also increase sleep deprivation. Experts agree that people experience higher rates of appetite and hunger when their sleeping time is limited.

But laboratory studies have shown that sleep-deprived people appear to eat far beyond their energy requirement, implying they eat for pleasure and reward.

Overall, the study results add further evidence to suggest that inadequate sleep plays a significant role in munching and appetite, the researchers said.

Although there is increasing data to show that not having enough sleep raises all forms of hunger, there is still the issue of if the opposite is also valid — specifically, if individuals get even more sleep, are they going to be less hungry?

Investigators have just begun to investigate the said question. Some research, for example, has shown that higher sleep time might reduce the feelings of hunger for certain foods. But till now, most of these "sleep extension" experiments have concentrated mainly on how blood sugar rates are influenced by sleep than on what foods people want and how frequently they consume. Therefore, to answer those questions, more research is required.

Exercise

The concept that workout can restrict appetite can sound counter-intuitive to anybody who's ever felt voracious upon working out. But some evidence shows that the amounts of hormones believed to control appetite that is reduced by some forms of physical exercise — including a fast, vigorous workout.

The appetite-inducing hormone ghrelin undoubtedly seems to be diminished by exercise. Exercise also tends to increase the rates of many other hormones, like cholecystokinin and peptide YY, which play a role in appetite inhibitors. However, more research is needed to exactly how exercise affects the reduction and trigger of such hormones.

But not all exercise kinds do occur to have some impact. Most people really feel hungry having done low- to moderate-intensity exercise, but for many individuals, this is the preferred choice of workout.

This seems reasonable that perhaps the body might well attempt to regenerate the energy is used in the workout, and after a workout, it is fairly easy to do this when the severity is comparatively low. In other terms, the body needs to consume food to offset the energy it just consumed, in order to regain health. But, by contrast, when someone performs a high-intensity exercise, the person undergoes much more metabolism changes rather than having lost calories. But while the body needs to regenerate its energy stores, before doing so, it highly values coping with certain other shifts.

All this raises the issue, will you actually exercise while experiencing the feeling of being hungry?

If the individual is hungry and had an exercise session of adequate duration, there might also be an advantage in minimizing hunger. Exercising at periods whenever you realize appetite seems to hit may also be an intriguing prevention choice, although this theory has not been discussed in a systematic study before.

8.4 Mind exercises for weight loss

Stay away from containers made of opaque material.

It is best not to consume out of food cans, bottles, and packets which are not transparent. The human brain is outstandingly conceptual. We take visual indications of how much food we have been eating to guide us to understand when we might stop. "But because you can't tell how much food you've eaten, you just have any tactile input, and you wind up consuming so much. Counting portions and dumping them into a cup or a napkin can deter you from consuming more than you've expected.

Review what you understand regarding losing weight.

The very first and best way to achieve one's ideal body is to understand weight loss in terms of an energy balance. Energy output and energy input is the way science says calories in vs.

calories out. Your body helps to keep its prevailing body weight within a certain number of calories. You can feel less motivated to consume more than you actually need because you realize the energy balance.

Abandon diet.

Calorie counting restricts one's mind-set. Once you're off your eating habits and lose weight, you may return to eating badly, not exercising, and ultimately regaining pounds. Rather, focus on your long-term eating habits. That's the key to weight loss and keep it off, a positive way.

Manipulate your tummy into satiation.

When you have a snack craving, it's advisable to choose vegetables like carrots and celery over sugar treats. They have fewer calories; they are also fibrous and can leave you feeling full quicker.

Be gentle with yourself.

You have to perceive yourself in a better light and break rid of old tendencies. Picture your hypothetical future, not far out from 6 months or even a year, and think how fantastic you can appear and sound.

Assume about exercising as having enjoyment.

Choosing a workout that is enjoyable helps the most, as you would be most inclined to integrate that into your everyday schedule. If you dislike running, don't run. It doesn't matter if running has been said to aid with weight reduction. Because you despise exercising too much, you won't stick to it. If you don't stick to it, it won't produce lasting results.

Motivate yourself by having to ask demanding questions.

Although self-assertions may be encouraging, try digging into the competitive side by making weight reduction into a competition. You may find it far more inspiring to motivate yourself with self-talking like this: 'Can you reduce this weight? Are you up for the test?

Find out what triggers obesity.

More incidents of obesity are reported to be caused by lifestyle choices instead of genetic and environmental factors. Trying to promote the concept of genetic makeup as a source of obesity can boost genetically probabilistic belief systems and reduce the desire to engage in healthy living attitudes. Individuals who believe that obesity is caused by unhealthy lifestyles are highly likely to be assertive and reconsider their behaviour.

Image Yourself Slim.

See yourself thin, because you would like to be slim. Envision your future self, down the path for six months to a year, and talk about how fine you'll look and sound without any of the extra lbs. Dig up your smaller self's old photos and place them in a spot as a sign about what you're working for. Question yourself whatever you knew back then, so now you might implement this into your life. Think of things you'd like to do, but because of your weight, you sure as hell won't.

Build a comprehensive Course of Action.

Each evening you prepare your next day balanced foods and workout. 80 percent of the struggle is looking ahead. If you are prepared with a comprehensive strategy, results will be seen.

Time your fitness as you would time for a booking. Pack dried fruits, vegetables, or food substitute bars, and you won't be forced to consume the poor types of food.

Make your healthy decisions by developing these actions into your life, and these positive habits will inevitably become the regularly scheduled part of people's lives.

Define your Small Targets.

Create a set of specific milestones to support you meet the expectations for weight reduction. Such mini-goals must be things that would make your way of life better without wreaking chaos in your daily lives, like:

• Eat the most from fruits and vegetables per day.

• Have a form of physical exercise for 30 minutes or more a day.

• consume beer on holidays only.

• Eat low-fat popcorn, rather than French fries,

• Order the side salad rather than the potato chips.

• Capable of going up a staircase without panting for air.

We all know change is difficult and, it's particularly hard if you're attempting to make too many adjustments, so start slowly and progressively implement changes in attitudes.

Set reasonable expectations.

When health care professionals question their clients what they'd like to weigh, the figure is always one that is feasible in practical terms. It corresponds to just 1-2 pounds a month, which would be completely doable, affordable, and achievable in the work and family sense. Within six months, you will be reassessing your fitness target.

Ditch aged lifestyles.

Old habits are difficult to quit, but if you want to succeed in losing weight, you can't keep on doing things exactly the way you had before.

Slowly but steadily, seek to find that you are involved in weight enhancing habits and transform them about with small actions that you can quickly manage without becoming drained off. If you're a lazy evening slob, for example, begin by shifting your meal from a packet of biscuits or fries to a slice of fruit. Try a calorie-free drink the next night. Inevitably, while watching TV, you can begin conducting workouts.

Another way to start digging your unhealthy habits: get rid of your kitchen's enticing, vacant-calorie food, and replace it with healthy alternatives.

Receive support and assistance.

We all need help, particularly during challenging periods. Find a mate, family member, or community network to whom you will frequently communicate. Studies show people who are connected to others, whether it's online or in-person, do smarter, unlike dieters who try to go at it alone.

Award Yourself.

Give yourself appreciation with a visit to the films, a pedicure, or something that can make you feel positive about your achievements (apart from diet rewards).

Incentivize yourself for achieving one of the mini-goals or having dropped 5 pounds or a couple of inches around the hip, and you recognize your hard work and acknowledge the efforts you make to be better.

Keep Record.

Weigh yourself regularly to keep journals describing in detail what you consume, how much you work out, what else you experience, as well as how much you weigh and assess. Studies suggest that holding this knowledge monitor tends to encourage good habits and reduce negative behaviours. Just knowing you're monitoring your calorie intake might help you withstand a certain slice of cake.

"Journals are a type of transparency that allows you to expose the methods that function. When you're responsible, you're less likely to get food disconnection or sleeping at the meal.

Chapter 09: Grasping Cheat Meals and Breaking Bad Habits by Training Your Mind

This last and important chapter gives insight into many things like a cheat meal, how to control it, and how to still choose within the healthy options. Take charge of your emotions to help prevent the binge eating and eating loads of processed food items. How you can overcome the negative behavior or habits is also discussed. Tips to make eating healthy automatic and natural are also discussed so that you do not have to worry prior to eating if eating healthy becomes your natural habit.

9.1 What really is a cheat meal?

Trying to cheat within the same eating plan means giving yourself scheduled, measured consent to partially drop fairly strict dietary regulations.

The idea behind such a reward-based eating approach is that you'll be more able to adhere to your standard diet much of the time while giving yourself short bursts of extravagance. Individuals will usually employ either a cheat food or a cheat-day strategy while using the cheat tactic. A cheat meal, as the term suggests, is a single food that deviates from your scheduled eating plan sequence, while a cheat day gives unlimited dietary choices for a whole day.

Options for cheat meals are extremely complex. How they are implemented might look quite different from person to person, based on the needs and targets of a person's eating habits.

Based on individual preferences, the decisions you make as cheat food would also differ from person to person, and they often come in the form of high-calorie foods that might not be allowed under a standard eating plan.

There really is no detailed advice regarding when or how invariably your cheat food or day must take place. People often will involve a single cheat each week, but this may probably depend on what the objectives for well-being or losing weight are for the individual.

The cheat tactic is versatile in this manner and can be enacted alongside a range of different diet patterns.

Remember that the cheat meal tactic is not suitable for all eating types. Some diets, like the keto diet, necessitate quite rigid compliance, without any room to cheat. The cheat strategy is, therefore, best used in diets that enable some adaptability.

Cheat food is planned meals usually contain extravagant food products that would not usually be permitted on your eating plan. A cheat day is anytime you give yourself a whole day to ingest whatever meal you desire.

9.2 How to keep it under control?

Cheat with plan

Planning is a critical component of a cheat diet. Prepare what to cook and what to eat. Many analysts believe one adjustment a week is enough at the peak. Lining up this big meal on a weekend or social event is a good idea. You know what you're going to consume by scheduling your cheat meal and can cut a few more additional calories previously throughout the day. It also allows users to find a favorite recipe in real terms rather than going to waste calorie intake with something you don't really like.

Use the toxin. Choose your spending spree, if you're planning on going out. Would you dive in carbohydrates, like a plate of bread or noodles, or chocolate cake? Or are you intending to toss a few alcoholic drinks back? Evict all three of these kinds of basic types from lounging at once. Focus just on one, including you will love yourself without going ballistic by holding the other types for another day.

Exercise Prior You Fest

Another way to reduce the cheat meal's fat benefits is to replenish the glycogen energy stores — the fuel in the blood that lights the body up with energy. How is it working? The body does not preserve carb as body fat till its stores of glycogen are depleted, meaning the roomier the reservoir, more and more space you have for, like, pasta until it falls on the legs. How are you going to do it? Before the unhealthy meal, visit the gym (ideally, before eating anything that particular day). Working exercises in the greater-rep exercise form are the perfect routines for exhaustion. It will create a difference with only 15 min. Need any additional boost? During your sweat-sesh, take a cup of black coffee. Studies show that caffeine, when chosen to take as a pre-workout substitute, can boost fat loss.

Get the Best kind of Cheat Meal.

Several cheat meals are better in comparison to others. And a moderate-protein, high-carbohydrate meal. Why? For what? Carbohydrates have the highest leptin effect, which helps you metabolize fat and feel content. And protein has the strongest impact on satiety owing to its effects on cravings-regulating hormones and strong thermal effect-the body's cycle of digestion of protein takes more energy than just about any other macro-nutrient. Would you like a role model? How about a pair of Sushi rolls? Steak, and a salad? Crepes and an omelet with eggs? And meatballs and spaghetti? .The options are practically limitless.

Request several other rounds

That is a couple of rounds of water. Fast foods generally have higher levels in salt, which hurls off anti-diuretic hormone levels — substances that regulate how often you pee — and can make you feel gassy and dehydrated. Start restocking the body when you drink in a couple of huge water glasses. Prior you hit the bed, and when you get up the very next day, fill those glass to drink with your meals. (And if you'd like to roll-start your hop back on the healthy eating ride, try incorporating in a couple of the finest teas for losing weight).

Get back on the right track.

"Everybody has the freedom to a cheat day, but none has the right to a cheat week—not especially on the birthday. 'Don't say, 'I've already compromised my diet, and I'm going to continue having anything I like.'" Enjoy your lunch and restart the healthier consuming routine as early as possible. "It would help you headed in the correct path and does not cause irreversible losses. White also suggests expelling the residue of the refrigerator to keep the cravings from attempting to reach you.

Emphasis on a single Cheat Plan

One approach that may help the culinary activities is to rely on only one or two unhealthy items, rather than attempting to incorporate all of them at one day.

Of starters, if you're preparing a cheat day, take only one or two of such extravagant choices instead of consuming the burger and fries, sweet drink, and desserts.

While concentrating your mind on the only single treat, excessively-consuming throughout your cheat time can make you least prone to tip the balance in quite an undesirable route.

However, though also changing the diet guidelines, you should start eating well and eliminating things that you realize you have trouble regulating around.

It could feel like a day where macro-nutrients or calories are not monitored, so you may indulge a dinner out without

thinking over what you pick from the list.

Such techniques may be particularly effective in diet situations for people who are having rough time self-control.

Development plan

For any big shift in the way of living, the secret to success is ready. When you have a good strategy in action, and the framework is designed to help you, you are less inclined to give in to the urge.

For cheat day or foods, certain people can find it challenging to recognize when to step on the brakes. Such an absence of self-control might actually make your dietary objectives less effective in the long-term.

Implementing a cheat-day schedule — much as you do on normal eating days — is a safe way to keep on board. It ensures that when you're encouraging yourself to eat things that you wouldn't usually eat, you should also retain charge of the process.

Of starters, it's a smart initial move to schedule where and when your cheat foods should be taking place. If you know you've got a birthday celebration and perhaps other social gathering heading up near the end of the week, planning your cheat food or day around with this occasion might be smart. You should always focus on maintaining portion sizes from there, even for more extravagant items.

Plan to get not more than one or two pizza slices for starters, instead of sitting in a chair for all the pizza.

Another strategy worth considering is to view the cheat day as an opportunity to pursue a regular, nutritious approach to meals by monitoring calorie intake and macro-nutrients. It provides you with a mental break from monitoring without exceeding the urge from any food.

Consider your regular diet pleasant.

A key factor to the explanation for diets are hard to sustain is that you don't want the meal you consume. Portion restriction and scheduled eating diet plans can be challenging to adopt on its own, so if you load that with stuff that you don't like, it will bring fuel to the flames.

Even because a meal is considered healthy does not really suggest you ought to consume it. Not to say, consuming things that you dislike is not a prerequisite to meet your targets for wellness and losing weight.

Integrating the things you love, and though you don't have a cheat meal or day, will be a perfect way to help your eating seem less like a burden. This will also enable you to retain better self-control over both eating and binge days.

Working for a healthy diet and lifestyle at the end of the day should be about creating positive improvements to suit your particular needs and desires — a no-size-fits-all solution exists.

When you can't handle this job on your own, suggest working with such a nutritionist or some other trained health care provider who will help you develop an efficient and fun diet program to meet your fitness goals.

Incorporating certain food approaches to cheat meals or events will further improve your desire to achieve your objectives. There are few ways of making a schedule for meal days, implementing healthy dietary habits, and choosing items you like on restriction times.

9.3 Make healthy eating automatic

Eat breakfasts forever

Breakfast is by far the essential meal of each day, indeed. Your body would accept breakfast after fasts in the night as just a way to improve the digestion and offer you stamina for a day

forward. Choose a nutritious breakfast low in unhealthy fats –
fruit-topped porridge, a milkshake, or protein loaded egg
whites are a good way to start the day with.

Have less processed food

Some of the smartest things to do with your eating is
consuming less refined foods. The refined products also
produce needless large amounts of sugar, fat, and salt. Taking
enough of an opportunity to prepare recipes from scratch
instead of consuming packaged foods. BBC Healthy Food is a
website filled with simple and easy meals to enable you to
know how to prepare your own meals.

Try looking things up to boost eating patterns

Just looking at the front of a food package is simple-particularly
for brands you've been acquainted with that for ages. What's
printed on the label's back, however, will tell a great deal
regarding the food you are consuming. When you can't figure
out what all of the components are, it's possible this isn't the
best healthy thing to consume. Search for basic, organic
ingredient products.

Consume fish two times per week

Oily fish is an essential aspect of a healthy diet, and consuming
at least two servings of fatty fish per week is

advised. Fish is delightful, low in calories, and loaded with omega-3, which also helps to maintain healthy heart conditions. Fish is simple to prepare, with rice or beans or even in chutneys.

Choose naturally bright products

Eating foods high in color are often abundant in antioxidants that offer defense towards various diseases, and this should be a compulsory part of the diet. Think of foods like green vegetables, lush berries, and vivid citrus to help you find to see which products you can consume.

Go one day per week, without meat

A day a week, going meat-free will allow you to consume more vegetables and fruit and offer you a change from such an animal flesh-heavy diet. There are some great vegan recipes out there, and consuming a vegan diet by spending in limit can be convenient. Why not pursue 'Mondays without meat' as a basic weekly guideline that the family members could follow?

Drink some more water

Not only does drinking water keep you hydrated, but it will also even make you feel better and avoid any desire to eat among meals. Have a glass on hand just in case, and you can drink consistently all day long and try to drink at least 2 liters on better offer the body everything it wants.

Pay heed to your body when it's hungry

Although keeping a watchful eye on your calorie consumption might assist you to eat healthily, skipping meals is not beneficial. Skipping meals could have a significant impact on your metabolic rate, and may cause you to overindulge later in the day to make up for your hunger. To help hold hunger at bay, many people consider it beneficial to consume five smaller meals throughout the day instead of three large meals.

Abandon sweet beverages

Sugar-filled drinks are a rich source of nutrient, less empty calories that, among other things, could affect your weight, oral health. Trying to cut out sugar-drinks is especially relevant to youth, but there are a few options that you might consider instead. Alcohol often has a strong sugar level, and while you are intoxicated, it's better going to the low-sugar alternative, or not consuming alcohol entirely.

Switch to Complex Carbohydrates

Whole-grain products must be an important aspect of the diet, and refined flour should be swapped out as much as reasonably possible. Foods like pasta, bread, couscous, and rice are all sold in variations of brown or whole grain and have a high content of fiber that makes them safer for absorption than refined foods. Here's why shifting to whole or multi-grain might improve well-being.

Healthier eating is a vital aspect of self-care, and implementing the basic guidelines about eating healthy will help maintain you on board.

9.4 How to overcome a bad eating habit

People are advised not to even call shifted food patterns a diet, which brings up all sorts of negative sentiments and perceptions, such as poverty, regulations, and food records.

It is important to speak about existing behaviors in terms of self-care when it comes to changing up unhealthy habits.

"Mindless snacking frozen yogurt each night can probably be described as negative conduct, but people do it to relieve or relax. So it's just self-care, and that just doesn't lead you somewhere far, but nevertheless self-care."

Seek to discover that you are doing such self-care behavior by telling oneself certain questions.

• If you eat the frozen yogurt at night, why?

- You're attempting to avoid what?

- What else are you keeping your attention away?

- Why do you have this urge to console yourself?

Once you more fully identify your causes, you could even initiate discussing the actual reason for the actions as well as breaking the bad habit. For example, "if you eat junk food each night and you're alone, how do you improve your social contacts?" Daniels says.

9.5 6 Ways to Handle Eating Bad Habits

Here are 6 strategies to help reduce the risk of your current, unhealthy behaviors and build sustainable ones:

1. Take the first small steps like a baby. Make minor improvements in your lifestyle and habits will boost your well-being as well as shorten your waistline. Any Professional recommendations:

- Begin a healthy breakfast every day.

- Get 8 hours of deep sleep per night because insomnia will contribute to overeating.

- Eat your meals sitting at a dining table, avoiding interruption.

- Eat the most food with family or partner.

- Teach yourself how to consume when you're starving and halt once you're full of contentment.

- decrease your quantity of food by 20 percent, or quit second shift.

- Seek dairy foods with lower fat content.

- Make whole-grain bread sandwiches and cover with mustard paste rather than mayo.

- Using strong caffeine and warm soy milk rather than cream to turn to coffee.

- Eat a snack or a balanced meal after a few intervals.

- Use non - stick cookware and cooking spray rather than oil to prevent the fats in dishes.

- Seek various ways of cooking, for example, roasting, grilling, frying, or poaching.

- drink lots of water and drink very little sugar drinks.

- Eat smaller amounts of calorie-dense products (such as pizza and casseroles) and greater amounts of fluid-rich foods

(like salads, broth-based soups, and veggies).

- Rather than just unhealthy sauces, savor the diet with spices, sugar, vinegar or lime

- Alcohol should be limited to 1-2 glasses each day;

2. Be More Conscious. One of the very first steps to conquer the poor eating habits is to pay more focus on what you eat and drink. Understand nutrition labels, get familiar with nutrition labels, and begin to note what you putting in your stomach. When you are more aware of what you consume, you will begin to understand how you ought to change your health. Many individuals profit from maintaining meal journal entries.

3. Create a clear plan; be precise. How can you continue consuming more berries, enjoying coffee each day, or exercising quite frequently? Entail out your possibilities. For instance: intend to take a slice of fruit to work for lunch every day, start stocking up on food and fruit for easy breakfasts and go to the gym three days a week on the way to or from work. "To claim 'I am willing to exercise more will not benefit you,'". "What's going to improve is to worry about where and how to incorporate it into your routine."

4. Every week, address a different small target. Such mini-steps ultimately add up to a big transformation. For instance, if your primary objective is to eat healthier, tell yourself that you are going to try one new veggie each week until you discover a few that you really like. Or search for simple ways to attach even another vegetable serving to the meal every week before you hit your target. Seek to add pieces of vegetables to your lunch sandwich; add sliced carrot to the cupcakes you have for breakfast, or finish off your pizza with sun-dried mushrooms and tomatoes.

5. Become Rational. Don't anticipate too much too fast of yourself. Any new action tends to take around a month to be a habit. Slowly and steadily earn the battle — including a dosage of watchfulness.

6. Managing distress. Concentrate on coping with depression by workout, therapy, reflection, or whatever helps you best, and at moments of tension, you don't slip back into certain unhealthy behaviors or using eating to assist and support you deal with the issue.

9.6 10 Steps to Change Negative Habits

1. Recognize the behaviors you really want to alter. This involves bringing your awareness about what is purely speculative (or at least disregarded). This isn't about picking yourself up for it. Write a number of items you want to alter and choose one.

2. See what you will get out of this. Or think of it another way, how does the behavior serve you? Searching for warmth in the food? Wine loss of sensation? An outlet or connection? Eating for stress relief or biting nails? This should not be a lengthy, complicated method. You're going to work things out — and you're going to get some interesting suggestions on how to change it on for better results.

3. Respect your own rationality. Here's a realistic situation: you seem like you don't have downtime, so you're staying up too late to see your absolute favorite Netflix show. You realize that the day after, you're going to be tired and less successful, so even for you, you feel "entitled" to doing something nice. Nevertheless, the intuition understands it was not a safe way to do it. Using the experience to create this into the routine that can truly produce whatever you want. Realize that you have the solutions, and are ready to pursue anything more.

4. To remove the bad habit, select one. Only trying to alter is just not enough, as it doesn't resolve the inherent value of the conduct you wish to substitute. What would you do while you are stressed, rather than queuing up next to the refrigerator? When you have a strategy, the resources and substitution actions should "power you." Consider a substitution action the next time you find yourself not starving yet staying in front of the fridge anyhow. Few ideas: inhale in at count 4 and exhale out at count 8, concentrating solely on the breath. Try it four times to see if you're doing okay. When you need further help, stay there before you show up of one argument why this practice does not continue. It is a critical move. When you try something new to cover a harmful practice, confess to yourself that you do it differently. You ought to put to the conscious awareness that it is that is latent, so you can reinforce the desire to alter. This can be as easy as saying, "Look at it. I really found a great decision.'

5. Turn away stimuli. When Doritos is a cause, toss those off on a day that you feel confident enough to do that. When you're drinking alcohol casually, and you want a smoke, stop external stimuli — eateries, pubs, evenings out with mates. This doesn't have to be forever — just for a while before in your new habit; you feel safe. Often, our causes are other individuals. Know you wind up looking, such as the five men you're always hanging out with. Look at who other individuals are: are they motivating you or pulling you down?

6. Envision changing yourself. Serious imaging helps to slow down the subconscious. For this situation, you would like to stay optimistic about your willingness to change — so invest some time each day, creating fresh patterns for yourself. Imagine yourself walking and loving it, consuming or slipping nutritious snacks into those pants. See you engaging in a comfortable discussion with others rather than stood at the rear of the room. This sort of simulation works very well. The already common theory of "nerves of burn wire together" is focused on the premise that the longer you think about it — and practice something — the more it gets installed in your head. In reality, your default option can be a better one for you.

7. Track your self-talk more towards the negativity. Your mind reserve will have a significant effect on your normal habits. And anytime you hear yourself thinking, "I'm obese" or "No-one likes me," redefine it or redirect. Re-framing is like story rewriting. Replace it with "I'm getting better," or "My confidence is improving." Redirecting is by introducing "I'm overweight" to the negative self-talk with "But I'm making my way towards a lifestyle change." Reassign the brain of judgment.

8. If possible, take small steps. Also, if you cannot carry upon a new practice at once, do anything little to hold you on board. Of starters, if you have scheduled out an hour of exercise and have to head to a doctor's appointment all of a sudden, find some way to get in at least 15 minutes. Yeah, you're trying to bolster your current practice, even though you cannot contribute 100 percent.

9. Understand you are likely to falter occasionally. We are all doing so. Behaviors will not move immediately — each time you do it and know that you are a person.

10. Know this is going to take some time. Behaviors usually shift over many weeks. To adjust the standard settings, you need to strengthen the array of nerves in the head.

Take the system within the consciousness by making notes. It's really easy to overlook a new strategy that's built with the highest motives but never improved. Take 15 minutes to prepare your good habit, pen in hand, to ensure maximum success.

9.7 It makes losing weight easy by rewiring the subconscious mind.

What Is Brain Training?

Training of brain works by referring to the Subconscious Mind. The subconscious mind accounts for 97 percent of our total brain activity and is accountable for our making decision, moods, cravings, and more.

Your subconscious is always alert yet still listening-even though it's not!

Your subconscious mind will trust when you use the correct terms and vocabulary to cause the constructive reaction required to achieve our objectives.

Brain training is a strong and efficient means of tapping into this knowledge to change the inner existence.

How and when to rewire your mental sub consciousness?

There are many methods you can manipulate and reconfigure your subconscious and your innermost values, and one of the most powerful is the usage of subliminal recording and one approach that is increasing in popularity.

Subliminal recording can have a notoriety for being a bit obscure, but it really is an easy idea. This operates on the idea of whispered constructive affirmations — but they are registered and transferred to a higher level of sound, and you don't perceive the words audibly — but they are heard by your sub consciousness at the edge of your consciousness and absorbed and retained as usual.

Through that process, the subconscious mind is slowly and spontaneously rewired from inside out, so much as having hypnosis or making optimistic affirmations, the adjustments last.

Especially hypnotism, in terms of weight reduction, can enhance the confidence that you will lose weight; they can help you feel better than this time around; it is for sure, you can adhere to the goals. They should sustain your enthusiasm for longer, make you love and looking forward to the workout, and strengthen your determination to help you overcome cravings and remain committed. Basically, they can begin to inculcate in you the kinds of values held by individuals who live healthily naturally, who have not been influenced by greasy food, or who love exercising.

If you have these kinds of values and ways of thought, your actions can improve, and you will eventually lose weight and be able to hold this off for good.

That's why this program does work, even though you don't!

The Subconscious Mind's processing power is 1 million times more effective than the Conscious Mind at affecting our habits. That suggests that teaching the subconscious to continue working toward your weight-loss target is much more successful than attempting to lose weight in the conscious mind.

Fact: Seeking to make progress by depending on the strength and pride being utilized by the Conscious Brain is like consuming just one drop of water because you're dehydrated.

Our Brain Learning Audios talk explicitly to brain regions, which build your life by performing 97 percent of the job. That's what really allows them to be so successful.

It is only by repeated episodes at deep subconscious rates that your ideal patterns will become entrenched and begin to manifest in your waking existence.

Preparing to train your sub consciousness is much Simpler than using your rational mind with willpower! This is why cognitive preparation is the key to reducing weight.

9.8 Daily Weight Loss Motivation with Mini Habits

1. Beware of the portions.

Many individuals eat approximately twice the average amount of meals consumed. Restaurants also deliver large servings, which will teach your mind to believe that the quantity of food the body requires is not beneficial to have hands-on the right serving proportions

2. Put the spoon down in between the bites.

It forces you to eat more gradually, which would be an easy calorie-cutting strategy. Whenever you take your time rather than snorting your meals, your body will naturally enroll the feeling of satiety that can take approximately 20 minutes to signal your brain. Plus, gradually eating will help the food to taste even better.

3. Gulp down water 24/7.

Although the body is basically a fairly smart tool, it can be vulnerable to slip-ups. "Sometimes, it is dehydration that triggers what you believe is a hunger pang. The" hunger "will lead you to snack because all your body requires would be some water.

4. Taking some time out to make lunch.

Not only can you save time by cooking your own lunch, but it can also make sure you exactly realize what you're putting in your body, so you get the correct foods. You're still less prone to miss lunch on busy days because you can only walk to the supermarket instead of trying to run out to purchase food. While missing those meals could help improve weight reduction, trying to deprive your body of regular meals will make you more likely to overeat it later.

5. Do not do anything else whilst you eat.

Focusing on food while there's stuff to do and viewing Instagram may be difficult, but munching away while you're disturbed will lead you to unintentionally indulge with more than you should. Disturbed food doesn't only create further intake at the time; it can also force you to consume further later in the day than is required.

6. Emphasize breakfasts.

"Eating a meal packed with healthy fiber and protein should keep you satiated, and will help you make healthier food decisions every day. Choose meals that are not carbohydrate explosions without something significant to hold you full, such as hash browns, warm cereal, and croissants, to maximize breakfast power. "Try poached eggs on the whole grain toast, simple Greek yogurt with a bowl of your preferred fruit, or a veggie-laden omelet.

7. Be a clever snacker.

If you're attempting to lose weight, snacking may be either your best friend or a potentially supportive, but undoubtedly manipulative saboteur. There's the problem of unknowingly getting in more than you thought, which you can remedy in a snap by pre-portioning the treats as per their portion sizes instead of only gnawing away at them willy-nilly. Another issue with snacking can rise if you eat without check throughout the day, rather than snacking mindfully. Check out the snacking habits for weight loss tips to make sure you are on the right path.

8. Sleep through adequate hours each night.

It may be tough to adhere to a healthy sleep schedule — especially while there are episodes of serial to catch up on — but having adequate rest is an effective way to promote weight loss. Sleeping helps maintain the hunger hormones leptin and ghrelin in control. Without an appropriate quantity, those hormones get unbalanced and may contribute to increased appetite.

9. Keep eating healthy as well on Sundays.

If you're infatuated with having eaten possibly the best

Monday through Friday but consider weekends an unrestricted-for-all food, you might not see the weight loss you're hoping. If you add it all up, trying to eat poorly and not exercising Friday through Sunday tends to come out to 12 days off a month. Instead of allowing weekdays to impact your habits, focus on achieving a positive lifestyle — with the occasional treat — that's feasible.

10. Concentrate upon small plates.

If you look at the same amount of food on a tiny plate vs. a big one, your eyes could tell you there's even more awesomeness on the smaller plate. That's because of what's known as the Delboeuf illusion, which demonstrates that wrapping everything with a lot of white space will make it seem bigger. Even though you don't consume enough, cutting down on the amount of plate area surrounding your food will drip your mind. However, doing its opposite may trigger your appetite by forcing you to think you only ate a little bit.

11. Scale back on eating in family style.

When you dine with serving dishes full of extra help right in front of you, you can slip into refilling your plate carelessly even if you're not still hungry. Instead, if feasible, restrict the meal on the table about what you're having to eat. Which is not to conclude seconds are strictly prohibited — just review in and see if you're still starving prior to actually getting back to reach a little more.

12. In restaurants, the seat faced away from the buffet table.

Seeing more food in your sightline will drive you into food-coma territory, particularly if you're trying to maximize the benefit of your money. Instead of eating when thinking for what you can reward yourself to next, turn your attention to the other food, and concentrate on just embracing what's on your dish. If you'd like more food once you're finished, the buffet would still be there.

13. Place vegetables up on the plate.

One of the easiest strategies to fall into a healthier eating routine is by introducing foods to the diet rather than cutting them. Failing to consume all of the beloved snacks will go end up backfiring in a spree, whereas gradually raising your food consumption will only produce positive results. "Not only are veggies packed with essential nutrients to keep the body balanced and energized, but they also provide fiber to makes you lean. Beginning small to prevent vegetable burnout: add a cup of them just to at most one meal per day for a week, and continue to integrate them into even more foods once you get accustomed to them.

14. Keep a diary of food.

If you practice any of these, but you don't see any significant weight reduction, it may seem like a complicated problem you really can't break. Keep a diet diary in any situation, such that you'll have a thorough and overall image of your behaviors. "It will help you identify places that are unique to both you and the habits that might use a little adjustment. Do the utmost and maintain control with the food and drink consumption for a whole week, and check out and see whether you are unintentionally getting in a few additional calories that you should leave out and achieve results you are seeking. Note, above all, that losing the weight always requires certain experimentation — but the idea is this is a long way you're practicing how to be healthy with the fitness, which really counts.

Conclusion

There are few simple and basic techniques or strategies that can be used to reduce weight in a healthy manner. Hypnotherapy among the others is getting popularity for weight reduction as it rewires the brain and nervous system, making it into thinking that the strategies being used are having a positive impact. Also, hypnotherapy is used for self-love, positive body image, and optimism for oneself. There is a complete guide on how to overcome negative thoughts and negative mindset. You can adapt the positivity, which will ultimately lead to better living. There are many other factors that lead to an unhealthy lifestyle, which has a drastic impact on human health and mind. To be physically fit, one should also focus on mental health as well. To divert your mind into positivity and optimism is a key to a healthy lifestyle. It will bring several other changes along with the health. It will help the individual to be more thankful, satisfied, and contented with his or her life. Eating and living a healthy and positive lifestyle should be incorporated in life in such a manner that it becomes natural and automatic for a person to always get attracted to healthy options or choices.

References

10 Ways Your Brain Is Making You Fat. Retrieved from **https://www.thehealthy.com/weight-loss/thoughts-and-weight-loss/**

12 Weight Loss Tips, Diet Plans & Weight Management Programs.   Retrieved   from **https://www.medicinenet.com/weight_loss/article.htm**

9 Proven Ways to Fix The Hormones That Control Your Weight.   Retrieved   from **https://www.healthline.com/nutrition/9-fixes-for-weight-hormones#section10**

Healthy   Weight   Loss.   Retrieved   from **https://www.cdc.gov/healthyweight/losing_weight/index.html**

How to Lose Weight Fast: 3 Simple Steps, Based on Science. Retrieved from **https://www.healthline.com/nutrition/how-to-lose-weight-as-fast-as-possible#1.-Cut-back-on-carbs**

How Your Body Fights Weight Loss. Retrieved from **https://www.nm.org/healthbeat/healthy-tips/how-your-body-fights-weight-loss**

HuffPost is now a part of Verizon Media. Retrieved from **https://www.huffpost.com/entry/weight-loss-psychology_b_881706**

Self-Hypnosis - Relaxation Techniques | SkillsYouNeed. Retrieved from **https://www.skillsyouneed.com/ps/self-hypnosis.html**

Weight Loss: How to Reset Your Brain For Success. Retrieved from **https://health.clevelandclinic.org/this-is-your-brain-on-a-diet/**

Weight Loss: Why Can't I Lose Weight?. Retrieved from https://www.medicinenet.com/weight_loss_problems_solutions/article.htm

PART 2

Deep Sleep Hypnosis

Introduction

Hypnotherapy has gained a ton of momentum in recent years, but especially in the popular culture. The science and medical professionals are just starting to acknowledge the real power of a hypnotic state. However, there have been many misconceptions and myths attached to the whole notion of hypnosis.

What comes to mind when you hear the word hypnotist? If you're anything like an average person, the name may conjure up images of a sinister stage-villain who creates a hypnotic state by swinging back and forth with a pocket watch. Apart from what you might expect, seeing a spinning wristwatch will not trigger hypnosis. In reality, it's the hypnotherapist's verbal signs that attract the hypnotized into an entranced state that can be easily demonstrated whenever you're so consumed in a novel book that you're turning off whatever is going on around you. For instance, an exercise that is designed to help you go deeper in your slumber would probably involve a gentle, soft sound, which would suggest that you're getting deeper, relaxing more, and falling asleep.

You will fall asleep afterward, or even while listening. Although some people interpret hypnosis as being incredibly calm, the brain is, in reality, concentrated on intense meditation during hypnotism.

Deep sleep hypnosis is likely to do wonders for certain types of individuals. It's because some individuals are much more prone to hypnotic suggestions than others, which means they get drawn more easily into an entranced state. However, roughly a third of people in the world simply cannot be hypnotized.

Hypnosis has become widely established due to popular acts in which individuals are persuaded to undertake odd or irrational behavior, but medical and therapeutic effects have also been clinically proven, most importantly in minimizing pain and anxiety. Hypnosis has also been proposed to reduce the symptoms associated with dementia. Although hypnosis is sometimes defined as a state of sleep-like trance, it is best articulated as a state marked by intense concentration, increased suggestibility, and vibrant fantasies. People in a hypnotic condition sometimes tend to appear being asleep and zoned out, when in reality, they are in a condition of hyper-consciousness.

Hypnosis, in general, shows no similarity to such traditional depictions in the popular belief. The hypnotist doesn't hypnotize the person. Instead, the hypnotist acts as a kind of mentor or teacher whose job is to help the person become hypnotized to achieve certain goals.

Hypnosis has been proven to show a plethora of benefits. It's a great and versatile therapy that has a wide variety of applications. Some of the things that hypnosis and specifically deep sleep hypnosis work wonder for include all kinds of addictions, e.g., cigarette addiction, alcoholism, binge-eating, opioids, etc. Furthermore, hypnosis also helps tremendously to resolve sleep disorders like insomnia, sleep-walking, sleep apnea, and night terror disorder. Also, sleep hypnosis has been proven to work well for improving low self-esteem by reaching and influencing the sub-conscious mind and re-framing the hidden belief in the background.

Therefore, in this book, we will talk about the different kinds of things that deep sleep hypnosis can be used to heal. First off, we will get into the detail of how hypnosis helps for overthinking, rumination, anxiety, and stress. Afterward, we will discuss how to use hypnotherapy to boost poor self-esteem. Then, in the next chapter, we will dive deeper into the Past Life Regression Therapy and how it is used to recover hidden past life memories and heal traumas. Moreover, one chapter will be dedicated to using hypnosis to quit smoking addiction. Finally, the book will end with tips and tricks to

enhance your self-hypnosis along with some information on
how to use a hypnotic gastric band for weight loss.

Chapter 1: The Basics Of Deep Sleep Hypnosis

In this chapter, we will talk about the basics of hypnosis and specifically about deep sleep hypnosis. This chapter will begin by defining what hypnosis is. Afterward, the stages of hypnosis will be discussed in detail. Then, we will move on to talk about the actual steps that a hypnosis session entails, whether it is self-hypnosis or a hypnosis session given by a professional hypnotist. Then, the first part will end with a detailed discussion of all the myths that have been associated with hypnosis over the last century since its inception by James Braid. Then, the second part of this chapter will entail an extensive discussion on the human subconscious mind, its structure and function, and how powerful it is in influencing our reality. Here, we will also get into the four major brainwave states which relate to sleep-wake cycles and hypnosis. Furthermore, we are going to look at the importance of a great hypnosis technique called auto-suggestion. In the next part, we will highlight the importance of deep sleep hypnosis for insomnia and sleep disturbances by relating it to brainwaves and how they help to induce hypnotic states in order to induce sleep. Finally, the last part of the chapter will highlight the benefits of deep sleep hypnosis for things like weight loss, smoking cessation, anxiety and depression, low self-esteem, and certain medical conditions like IBS, arthritis, and related pain management and heartburn, etc.

1.1 Defining Hypnosis

Hypnotherapy is the introduction of a sleep-like coma condition, in which you become particularly vulnerable to hypnotist intervention or guidance. You reach a condition throughout hypnotherapy, where you become more centered and prepared to focus. The hypnotherapist allows you to unwind and settle down while allowing you more responsive to advise. Hypnotherapy is similar to fantasizing. If you have a fantasy, you appear to ignore all personal emotions or distractions and only concentrate on your fantasy.

You are also driven throughout hypnosis to concentrate entirely on what's occurring in the present moment, while not getting disturbed by any emotions or noises. In this way, the subconscious in the entrancing condition is particularly sensitive to suggestions. That's why hypnotherapy is so strong.

Hypnosis is a behavioral condition of extremely intense attention, reduced sensory perception, and greater suggestivity. Professionals utilize various strategies for causing such a condition. Doubling down on the influence of persuasion, hypnotherapy is also used to make individuals calm, reduce stress sensitivity, or promote a necessary improvement of behavior.

Hypnotherapy is, in the easiest words, a calming method where participants adopt procedures to achieve a condition of enhanced focus and calming. That is considered the "hypnotic condition," so it's close to fantasizing, or the sense of losing count of hours you get when traveling for lengthy spans of the period (which is labeled "road hypnosis").

Therapists carry in hypnosis (also known as hypnotherapy or entrancing statement) with the aid of visual visualization and a calming vocal voice that ease the individual into a trance state. Upon recovery, the brains of clients become much more accessible to positive communications.

You are kept alert and in charge during the hypnotherapy. Yet you are incredibly confident and concentrated. It helps you to change sensations surrounding you and achieve an enhanced level of consciousness.

Two key components in hypnosis are activation and suggestions. Trance-like initiation is the very first instruction offered during much of the hypnosis process, though it is still a question of controversy on what it will consist of.

Typically, suggestions are presented as consequences that cause apparently unconscious reactions from individuals that may not feel that they have any or little influence (or authority) throughout the scenario.

Several individuals are often more "suggestible" than the others, and studies find that extremely impressionable persons are more likely to be under a trance and have a decreased sense of control.

Trance-like suggestivity is characterized as "the capacity to notice proposed improvements in perceptions, sensations, feelings, ideas, or actions.

You may think of hypnosis as targeted meditation. These are related in that you'll strive to achieve a state of calm and focus. But you can push that a level better through hypnotherapy. You continue to explore the subconscious in this condition of elevated consciousness, and you are presented with feedback that will help to change, strengthen, and reinforce the way the subconscious works.

Hypnosis-induced suggestivity may act to alleviate chronic depression. Hypnosis is often used to cure other medical problems, such as stomach diseases, skin diseases, or severe discomfort, but, naturally, hypnotic therapy is not effective in all instances. Hypnosis was often utilized by psychologists to gather knowledge regarding its effect on thought, memory, experience, and interpretation.

Reports also have shown that hypnotherapy can alleviate the effects of IBS in the short term, although it has not yet been definitively checked for long-term efficacy.

Sleep disturbances and insomnia can also be fixed with deep sleep hypnosis. Hypnosis may also treat anxiety, hallucinations, and night-time terrors (which appear to impact adolescents aged 7 to 12), as well as certain more severe sleep disturbances, such as sleepwalking. Comments for relaxing and ego-control are also used to resolve certain situations.

Some evidence shows that hypnotherapy may be helpful in managing migraine headaches and anxiety attacks, and because of the absence of adverse effects, it may be good alternate therapy.

Extensive research by the Center for Holistic and Multidisciplinary Health indicates that hypnosis may benefit patients who like to quit smoking, particularly if combined with other recovery approaches. Yet convincing proof in this scenario, too, is ambiguous.

It is a condition of trance marked by severe suggestivity, stimulation, and heightened creativity. It's not about sleep, though, since the topic is warning all the time. It's more commonly related to fantasizing, or the sensation in a movie or show of "losing oneself." You are well aware of this, however much of the sensations surrounding you are tuning out. To the complete absence of all other thinking, you concentrate deeply on the topic at hand.

In the ordinary trance of fantasy or video, an imagined universe appears to you to be very real, in the way that it activates your feelings entirely. Imaginary things may trigger genuine terror, sorrow, or joy, and if you are shocked by anything (for example, a creature jumping out of the shadows), you can jolt into your seat. Any scholars describe both of those trances as types of self-hypnosis.

In classical hypnotherapy, you follow the hypnotist's ideas, or your own feelings, as though they were fact. When the hypnotherapist says your mouth has swelled up to double normal height, you may experience pain in your jaw, and you might be experiencing difficulty communicating. If you're consuming a glass of milk, the hypnotist advises you to taste the glass of milk and sense it relaxing the mouth and neck. When the hypnotizer indicates you're afraid, you can become jumpy or begin sweating. Yet all of the ways, you know it is all fictional. Just as children do, you pretend to an emotional stage.

Individuals feel unrestrained and comfortable in a unique psychological condition. It is probably that they iron away from the fears and suspicions that usually hold the acts in control. While reading a book, you may encounter the very same impression: When you get immersed in the story, concerns about your career, friends, etc. melt away before all you're worried about is what's in the book. Most people are extremely impressionable in this setting. That is, if the hypnotherapist asks you to do it, then you would possibly totally accept the notion.

Hypnotherapy is a very healthy procedure commonly accepted by science and medical professionals as a tool that can transform lives in a meaningful way. Whether you are better, happy, more trust, and less tension in life, therefore the solution is hypnosis.

The hypnotic influence happens when an individual becomes so deeply concentrated that it causes the subconscious mind's limitless capacity to function beyond the rational mind's imagined limits, culminating in emotional and psychological improvements.

It is worth noting that hypnotherapy was being used for decades, but it was not eluded to back then as hypnosis. In reality, it wasn't until the late 1800s that a Scotland surgeon, James Braid, coined the term "Hypnosis" from the Greek term 'Hypnos' meaning sleep.

James Braid is generally recognized as the first hypnotist and was credited for elucidating and making hypnosis more available. Until Braid's research, there was a widespread misconception that this method of therapy succeeded due to animal magnetism and magnetic fluid transfer.

James Braid quickly disproved this hypothesis of animal magnetism and then found that only four simple laws had to be observed in order to trigger a trance-like state. These steps are:

Step 1

The first rule is to catch the attention of the client. To accumulate information, you only want to catch the client's interest and concentration. This included communicating and interacting with the customer in a way that attracts clients to you, leveraging the tonality, psychology, and reputation, to make sure that perhaps the customer is able to obey your orders. When you have this done, you step on to step 2.

Step 2

The second step is to tame the rational mind. The vital part is the portion of the brain that does not believe and utilizes rationality and justification. When you've ever seen a show, and you've been commenting on how those details aren't physically possible – that's your critical part of the brain.

All hypnotherapy is self-induced, and by removing their skepticism, you would like to help the client to eliminate their aversion to a hypnotic state. This helps the client to take an involuntary reaction to you. Having bypassed the vital faculty, the brain becomes more open to hypnotic ideas and symbols. But if a patient is disturbed in a visit, or is worried for their safety, the Important Faculty of the patient turns immediately back on, disrupting the entrancing state.

Step 3

Unlocking subconscious thoughts is the strongest indicator of a good therapist bringing the individual into a trance-like state. An indication of a subconscious reaction is a neural reaction to which is not produced consciously. There are forms of reactions that are generated at the implicit stage and often arise without a person being mindful of them.

A strong illustration of these forms of involuntary reactions can be observed. For instance, the client's salivary glands are activated in reaction to imagining them chewing on a lime, or a noticeable twitch as the customer envisions the sight of fingers scraping down aboard. Such outward representations are the result of the subconscious mind that reacts to the emotions and visualizations you are helping the customer to construct.

Step 4

The final step is to direct the mind to the ideal result. Hypnotic ideas & symbols should be utilized once a person is in an entrancing condition, and the hypnotist has supported the person to reach the three preceding phases effectively. Usually, hypnotic ideas are used as orders, which may be used to establish instantaneous impact or post-hypnotic results. Metaphors are tales deliberately designed and transmitted to make the subconscious mind be more industrious, creating a more favorable outcome.

When a hypnotherapist effectively integrates all four phases, both patient and the therapist participate in a hypnotic experience, which results in the client being more resourceful when solving their problems and challenges.

Stages of Hypnosis

Hypnotherapy always starts with planning or screening a map for the therapy. Hypnotherapy treatment is typically performed in a quiet, comfortable, secure atmosphere clear of interruptions. The initial chat between the individual to become hypnotized and the hypnotist usually outlines (if any) perceptions and previous hypnosis experiences. In fact, the particular issue that needs to be focused on is addressed. Sometimes these areas of concern include habits or beliefs which have to be changed; or entirely modified. For starters, assist with cigarette cessation or fat loss.

You may not undergo hypnosis with a hypnotherapist or psychologist during your first visit. Alternatively, you two might chat about your goals and the method they might use to assist you.

Your doctor can make you calm in a relaxed environment during a consultation on hypnotherapy. They will describe the process and will study your session goals. They would instead use repeated vocal cues to direct you through the condition of trance-likeness.

If you are in a trance-like state of receptivity, the psychiatrist will recommend you strive on those objectives, help you envision the life, and direct you on making better choices. Your therapist will then terminate the trance-like state by ushering you back to conscious awareness.

A professional hypnotist learns a lot of knowledge during the initial chat. Therefore the introductory chat should allow the hypnotherapist to figure out a single individual's effective induction strategy.

Following is the outline that is followed:

1. Planning or screening of the problem

2. Induction of enhanced state of trance

3. Deepening of the condition of trance. This is proven to increase the level of impressionability.

4. The post-hypnotic suggestions. The suggestions are offered on the question or region in the subconscious to be focused on.

The method is composed of several phases:

1. **Induction**: You must go through the whole phase, called the

entrancing induction, to achieve hypnosis. In fact, with eyes shut, you'll be sitting on a chair (or sitting on a sofa, bed, or relaxed anywhere). Regulated relaxation exercises and/or a template may also be used to calm and concentrate. Individuals may obey a rehearsed template, a tape, or a skilled hypnotist may trigger them.

Usually, the very first 15 minutes are intended to calm the body and mind in a hypnosis procedure. The first hypnosis stage is named the induction. The phases of induction involve urging a participant to use calming methods to reach a 'warm trance.' These forms of calming work both for the body and the mind.

The method of gradual induction allows the individual to be hypnotized to concentrate on all their muscles and calm them. In fact, this method of physical calming helps get rid of the stress and relieve fear. Typically some focus is paid to calming down and regulating the breath; this, again, facilitates relaxing and diverts the rational brain. There are various different methods of induction, and various people can respond to some better than the others. Hence, a highly personalized method of hypnotherapy treatments is critical.

Many people want to do something to calm mentally until the introduction phase of hypnosis therapy, including having a hot Jacuzzi with herbs or relaxing to classical music. You take a relaxed and calming posture throughout the hypnotic induction phase, too, and shut your eyes. Lying on a couch or on the floor is normal, but if you choose to sit up straight, then this will function as well. Most of the induction is to ready yourself to join the trance, and another way to get your body and mind going is to breathe deeply in and out.

You could breathe in for counting of five, for e.g., and breath out for counting of six. Most individuals find it beneficial to have an application that presents a calming picture between inhalation and exhalation directions.

Many hypnotists often provide a template which will direct you through this initial relaxing point. You may also attempt to compose your entire version or modify the one you've already used if you're more qualified.

2. **Trance Condition**: You enter the entrancing condition during an induction. You feel emotionally and psychologically comfortable in a trance-like state, you are quiet and concentrated, and you perceive an increased awareness.

In this stage, you reach the hypnotic trance itself. As mentioned before, this is an extremely comfortable and highly open form of life. It is the phase when the subconscious should be open to accept ideas that encourage constructive progress. Rather than fewer, you will be much more conscious of the environment, so you'll be able to shift clear attention to anything you want. You'll be using this emphasis to refine whatever you need to learn or alter for yourself.

Your body is probably going to be incredibly comfortable, and the muscles may seem relaxed and heavy too. A feeling of peace permeates, and that is what many individuals might find fun. Hypnosis will also enable you to alleviate fatigue in conjunction with promoting improvement.

3. **Hypnotic Suggestion**: The client gets entrancing feedback while he is under hypnosis. Such ideas are for removing and modifying your unconscious feelings. Suggestions can be presented in different ways. Conventional hypnotherapy uses clear orders, while metaphors are used by classical hypnosis. On the other side, NLP uses suggestions that strongly imitate our modes of thinking.

The third phase of the trance-like phase is the expansion of the state of trance. This 'deepening trains the subconscious mind for fresh ideas to be more open. Additionally, different forms of thought and actions can occur since the latest ideas are implemented.

Often the methods used to intensify the state actually go on and strengthen the form of initiation selected. However, these approaches typically require a strengthening of body stimulation along with the hypnotist-led in-depth imagery strategies. Securing that the subject has reached a 'strong' condition of enhanced awareness is quite important; before going on to the process's 'hypnotic suggestion' level.

The next step of the hypnotic cycle is the suggestions meant to alter habits of thinking and behavior. Perhaps the hypnotist would have decided these ideas for self-improvement, as well as the individual in the original presentation. It is really necessary to phrase the suggestions in a positive way. Evidence has found the unconscious mind is reacting well to such ideas in a trance and doesn't give critical feedback.

A professional hypnotist should be able to formulate the ideas in such a way that each person can react to the transition. The suggestions do need to be presented in a way that matches well with the subject's 'worldview.' Throughout the hypnotic process, a post-hypnotic suggestion is made. Yet it will have an impact on the future at a later stage.

Additionally, a suggestion should be acknowledged automatically. Yet the argument would have to be replicated more frequently over many days to find a hold in the unconscious mind. When the idea takes root, however, habits of thinking will continue to shift. Finally, the latest forms in behavior contribute to significant improvement in behavior. Post-hypnotic feedback may be either visual or audible-; t depends on each person and how they react to the environment.

A successful hypnotist can determine how responsive an individual is to visual and auditory stimuli in the preparatory or 'screening' process. Additionally, extra physical hints may be offered as the hypnotherapist directs a topic from a trance of light into a trance of 'deepening.'

While you're in a hypnotic state, the recommendation stage begins. At this level, you are getting signals that help transform the subconscious thinking and motivate you to improve the ways you like. Specific methods of hypnosis have various forms of delivering these ideas. Traditional hypnotherapy, for instance, requires instructions (e.g., "You are feeling positive" or "You don't want to drink anymore"), whereas more conventional approaches may utilize symbolic pictures or less straightforward advice.

For starters, a technique called NLP Planning lets you imagine how you can reach the next occasion you activate the pattern of self-doubt. It is a means to get the responses to be re-shaped. Some approaches insert hypnotic ideas in longer phrases to enable the thinking mind to counteract the ideas.

When the suggestions are produced and fully accepted, you are advised to escape gradually from the trance-like state and revert to your usual consciousness form. It's important to do so gradually and softly, because the sudden release from a trance-like state may seem startling.

Myths about Hypnosis

Unlike popular belief, you can't be forced to cluck like a chicken. You take measures for your own desire. Know that hypnotherapy is not a magical mechanism of the mind. Rather, it is analogous to sleep. You take measures that enable you to reach a profoundly focused and peaceful state, and you stay in charge.

As mentioned above, when discussing hypnosis, it's normal to think about your rights and autonomy. So it is important to be specific on what is not hypnosis. Perhaps notably, videos typically portray hypnosis, demonstrating a means of taking influence over others. In reality, there's nothing hypnosis will make you do something you don't like.

You maintain the sense of your environment during, for one

aspect, and you can stop the cycle at any moment. You are not unconscious, so the concentration during the hypnosis is still heightened. Perhaps worth mentioning is that hypnosis does not require any special treatment, and you won't be sedated physiologically.

Third, you're not prone to ideas that aren't in accordance with your general beliefs and priorities, and no one may use hypnosis to transform you into another human or have you behave in ways that go against your will. Hypnosis is about shifting behaviors and emotions that don't fit for you, allowing you to grow into your own true selves.

Your subconscious mind is thirty thousand times stronger than your conscious mind. Some people often feel insecure about the prospect of losing influence, believing they can reveal information against their will. Yet note that you're actually incredibly relaxed — you won't say something you wouldn't usually reveal. When someone wants to question or say something that makes you upset, you'll only escape from hypnosis and be free to get out of the problem.

Sadly, the reputation of hypnotherapy has been tainted by mass media and certain crazy stereotypes put in. Popular examples are the following: You lose control: Hypnotized individuals learn their environments to the max. And reach a more focused degree. We wipe out noise, ease, and settle the subconscious. There's no lack of power, though. Anytime, you should raise your door.

Another misconception is that you are unaware or sleeping. During hypnosis, the intense concentration and relaxation experienced are frequently confused for sleeping or unconscious. This is why the term hypnosis originates from the old Greek term "hypno" or sleep. However, unlike sleeping, you are awake and fully aware of that.

Some believe that in hypnosis, you might get trapped. You see it in film-for the first moment anyone attempts hypnosis, but they don't ever wake up. We stay forever, hypnotized. But that's pure fantasy. You are all in charge; you can reopen the eyelids and return to your world.

Sure enough, you might have asked whether, in a hypnotic trance, it's possible to get "stuck." This is a terrifying thought, akin to experiencing a coma. Happily, regardless of the degree of influence you have over the condition that is again unlikely. No one at a hypnotherapy appointment has ever been caught in a trance. You will definitely come out of the hypnotic trance at any moment you like, and re-engage completely with the surroundings.

Finally, one common misunderstanding people have regarding hypnosis is that with limited intervention, it will heal or change almost every type of depressive thought. However, to assist with hypnosis, you have to decide to improve it, so it doesn't negate the desire for potential success, so productive development. It also allows you to keep up with your objectives, shift your values, and to increase your inspiration.

Hypnosis is usually seen as magic, which is not true. Hypnotherapy does not constitute a remedy. You need to be willing to make a change, so you have to keep focusing on it. Yet research has proven hypnosis will benefit if you really want to be better.

Individuals frequently dread that being hypnotized will cause them to lose control, surrender their will, and become dominated by them, but a hypnotic state is not the same as gullibility or weakness. Many people who base their hypnotic assumptions on stage activities yet fail to consider that stage magicians preview the participants to select those that are willing to cooperate, with possible exhibitionist tendencies and responsive to hypnosis. Stage activities continue to establish a hypnosis misconception that discourages people from searching for genuine hypnotherapy.

Many think that people are not in charge of their bodies while they are hypnotized. Through hypnosis, you are completely in control of the body. Given what you see with fake hypnosis, you should be conscious of what you do and what you have been told about. If you don't choose to do things that you are told to see during hypnotherapy, you are not going to do so.

Another misconception about hypnosis is individuals losing consciousness and getting amnesia. A small percentage of subjects going into very deep trance levels will fit that stereotypical image and have spontaneous amnesia. Most people have in mind everything that happens in hypnosis. This is useful since most what we'd like to fulfill in hypnosis can be accomplished in a trance of medium depth, where people tend to remember all.

During hypnosis, the subject is not under the hypnotist's influence. Hypnosis is not something that people have forced on them, but what they do by themselves. A hypnotist basically helps to direct them as a facilitator.

While hypnotherapy is gradually becoming more recognized in western medical practice, there are still many myths about hypnosis. Here we distinguish truth from lies.

It's a myth that everybody can be mesmerized. One research

shows that only 10 percent of the world is extremely hypnotize-able. While the majority of the populace might have been hypnotized, they are less likely to be susceptible to the procedure.

A myth is that hypnosis is the same as sleeping. You appear like you're dreaming, but during hypnosis, you're alive. You are literally in a state of intense relaxation. The limbs get lax, the respiratory speed drops, and you can feel drowsy.

One belief is that when entranced, individuals cannot lie. Hypnotherapy is not a serum of reality. Though during hypnotism, you become more willing to take advice, you do have the independent will to choose moral judgments. Nobody will force you to say something-fib or not-you don't want to admit something.

A myth is that several mobile devices and internet videos advocate self-hypnosis, but they are actually unsuccessful. This is not true. Self-hypnosis can work equally well.

Scientists in 2013 discovered that an accredited hypnotherapist or hypnotherapy institution typically does not create such tools. Experts and psychotherapists warn about utilizing them for this purpose.

1.2 Subconscious Mind – Its Structure And Functionality

It is thought that by the time you reach the age of 21, you have already processed the details of the whole Wiki Britannica more than a hundred times indefinitely.

Through hypnotherapy, elderly persons are still able to recall incidents occurring 50 years ago, with complete accuracy. Their implicit recall is nearly fine. Accused is the active recollection.

The subconscious has the task of saving and retrieving info. The role is to make sure you answer as you're configured. The subconscious mind is making what you say to suit a template aligned with your "master plan" self-concept. That's why reinforcing optimistic affirmations are so efficient – you can literally re-wire all your ways of thought by sliding into constructive to ambition-oriented sound bites.

That explains how motivating practices are particularly meaningful for individuals dedicated to healthy thought, like hearing inspiring quotations. Through concentrating your attention on elevating concepts, your unconscious can start introducing a constructive trend in your mindset and life outlook.

The subconscious thoughts are subjective. It does not autonomously believe or justify; it simply follows your aware mind's instructions it continues to receive. Much like your rational mind can be seen as the gardener planting seeds, so can your subconscious mind be seen as the greenhouse or fertile soil where the seeds grow and expand. This is yet another explanation of why it is essential to channel the influence of happy thought to the base of the entire cycle of thought. It is the job of the conscious thought to rule, and the inner self complies.

The subconscious mind is also an undisputed agent who operates day and night to make the actions align with your emotionalized feelings, dreams, and wishes. In the garden of your existence, your subconscious mind develops either roses or weed, which you plant through the mental parallels you make.

The subconscious mind does what is recognized as a homeostatic drive. It holds your core temperature at 98.6 Fahrenheit; it maintains you are inhaling steadily at a certain pace and prevents your heart pounding. It ensures equilibrium amongst the millions of substances in your trillions of cells across your autonomous nervous system, such that the whole physical body can work in total harmony much of the time.

In your internal domain, the subconscious still maintains homeostasis by holding you thought and behaving in a form that is compatible with everything you have accomplished and expressed in the past.

Many of your thought and behavior patterns are contained inside your subconscious. It has all your comfort bubble memorized, and it helps to keep you inside them. That is why it's so important to make a daily habit of writing SMART goals. Staying successful and concentrating on all of your priorities should become a component of the comfort bubble over time.

The subconscious triggers you to feel psychological and body-wise insecure any time you want to do something fresh or different, or to alter some of your existing behavior patterns. The feeling of terror and anxiety are mental indications which are triggered by your subconscious. But it's been focusing on creating such habits of actions in the past well before you would even experience these feelings.

Another explanation of why routines can be too challenging to shake is the urge to stick to certain trends. However, as you begin to build these habits consciously, you will manipulate

the force of habit and deliberately inculcate new personal boundaries that your subconscious can respond to.

Each time you attempt something different, you can sense the subconscious dragging you back into your comfort bubble. Just talking about something which is special from what you've been used to doing can make you feel nervous and anxious.

That's why time management advice may be harder to adapt initially, but they might remain in your comfort zone once they are habit or schedule. You re-wired your mind in doing so to function to your advantage.

Successful males and females still reach out and force them off of the comfort bubble. They are very conscious of how easily the comfort zone becomes a rut in any environment. Cynicism is the biggest adversary of imagination and the prospects of the future.

Before you to evolve, you need to be prepared to feel insecure and nervous, trying new stuff the first several times and move outside of the comfort bubble. If it's worth doing well, then it's worth doing badly once you get a feel for it, before you build a new comfort level at a different, higher level of ability.

The subconscious becomes the ego fully unseen. Completely no one can sense their subconscious at play, because we don't have some way to tell what the latest feedback is really being correlated with, that explains why we might unexpectedly hate a single person or even encounter a burst of anxiety for any fairly minor occurrence. Of furthermore, it can function in reverse almost as effectively; if you ever have the case when you want things so much that it sometimes confuses you, and then you'll know. And then, you say things such as: "Just Goodness understands why I'm so addicted!" No matter what it is, it may be a peculiarly offensive friend, or perhaps a fashion object or almost everything.

Perhaps that is a little difficult to take on the deck, but it is a reality that by the time you become cognizant of a sensation, an input from all of the senses, even your own mechanisms of thought, by the time you become aware of that stimuli, the subconscious has detected it, checked it several hundred times, and had already decided to initiate an intervention dependent on that. And the thinking mind interferes, and that's the root of confrontation in summary. The subconscious encourages you to undertake any or any activity that is separate from what you actively intends to do.

A sign, in the sense of our mind's internal processes, is nothing but a trend of conduct that is disproportionate to the condition we often identify ourselves in. A perfect example is a phobic reaction – there's typically no clear reason, but the anxiety it may produce is overwhelming. Often, these signs are nothing but an established pattern, a programmed reaction, no matter what they would be. And even that does have its origins in subconscious systems, or we'd all avoid doing something that's. Or continue doing everything we say we can't.

The subconscious has little justification or reasoning, little judgment or critique, no requirement, or allocation. Anything in the subconscious is black or white, either it is, or it is not. It is, in essence, nothing but a responsive emotional core whereby the intuitive abilities live, both those with which we were born and those with which we have gained over the life cycle. For each and every fraction of a second of our lives, it is an evaluation process that continuously takes up every possible input via our sensations.

The subconscious communicates only through feelings with the aware mind, and it utilizes that interaction to try to keep us safe. It seems like any new feedback through the five senses can be measured against all we have seen so far in our existence. If the new feedback fits something that has already been done, so the response that we have would focus on the outcome, be it a positive response, which may be enjoyment or a negative reaction that maybe anxiety.

The bad part regarding the subconscious is it doesn't offer an opportunity to deliberately rationalize our direction about what it really does because it interacts with us only through feelings that regulate our responses. If through rational thinking, we seek to resolve certain feelings and emotions; therefore, the subconscious spurns its attempts! Have you ever attempted to justify anxiety because the aware mind is unable to understand why the apprehension is in reality there first? Stage fright is an outstanding example of this kind of thing. Some individuals have unreasonable public-speaking anxiety, but what would really take place anyway? Okay, you could make a mistake and maybe miss what you were about to do, but the dried mouth, leg-shaking, stomach-upset, heart-racing sensation of true panic that can always occur in just talking about it is a little 'over-the-top,' if done rationally! But this doesn't all go anywhere when you recognize it. The subconscious 'studied' the response, kept it on deck as an impulse intended to help defend you, and now have no intention of having you make any improvements to it. This cycle is almost definitely related to our primitive processes of survival through our pre-human times, hundreds of thousands of years ago. It is exactly because it has already been perceived by the subconscious that we will need the meaningful response for subsistence that it has already been confined to a location in our mind where conscious thought does not need to operate, and consciousness cannot interfere with it, well we almost cannot.

1.3 How Sleep Hypnosis Works?

In reality, an Austrian doctor called Frances Mesmer – after whom the word mesmerize is called – first worked with bringing clients into just a trance-like condition starting in the 1770s. Mesmer will play exotic jazz, fade the lamps, and also use methods for relaxing.

Yet Mesmer also had eccentric feelings on what was going on whilst in sleep; that is, he was injecting intangible electrical fluids to patients. Despite Mesmer's conclusions being incorrect, he has ignited our mutual interest in the area of hypnotherapy.

Today, when in a hypnotic state, there have been two major fields of thinking about what is happening in mind. The state-theory of hypnotherapy argues that people under therapy reach an abnormal state of mind. Such topics can detach perceived behavioral power from consciousness in this unconscious state. Subjects will ignore important cognitive thinking and concentrate on what they are doing before knowing why.

For starters, Ernst Hilgard had participants holding their hands in a bucket of ice water in an early hypnosis trial. Compared to un-hypnotized participants, anyone under hypnotherapy was willing to keep the palms in the fluid for way too long; yet in the end, as the pressure was too intense, they left the state of trance and withdrew their hands.

How Hilgard's analysis shows is that even undergoing hypnosis, participants were able to ignore rational thinking – "this liquid is freezing." Because that's what the state hypothesis suggests: that while regular brain functions are disrupted, we enter a state of intense relaxation.

The non-state hypothesis of hypnotherapy, In contrast, the non-state theory assumes that mesmerized subject plays a person's role under hypnosis. We have certain expectations and conclusions about how we are supposed to behave in this position, and that affects our actions even during a session of hypnotherapy. Positive reactions to hypnotherapy are then established as this is how the participants hope or believe that they will behave afterward.

One might ask, "Which hypothesis is telling the truth?" The

latest work shows that the hypothesis of the state can possibly be right. Work has demonstrated that brain activity improves while operating on mesmerizing ideas due to the new neuroimaging techniques.

And the inquiry seems to be quite convincing. Here's one example: Dr. Amir Raz, a professor at Columbia, requested clients to perform a basic task in 2005. Four words in block letters were written-GREEN, BLUE, RED, and YELLOW. But with each, the color of the ink used was incompatible with the written term. For example, red ink could have been BLUE.

Our minds would naturally choose to tell blue whenever questioned what hue the term Blue is printed in, even if the right response is purple. This is also regarded as the Stroop Effect, i.e., those incompatible thoughts are crossed, and we need to comment for longer.

Dr. Raz, therefore, hypnotized the participants and instructed them that on a computer, they will see terms in word salad, and the job was to recognize the ink color. Not only did the entranced participants perform the assignment without interruption, but brain imaging was not used to stimulate the part of the brain that transcribes written language.

In other experiments, patients have shown color pictures as black and/or-and-white, with a very corresponding impact on the region of the brain that detects inactive light. Such, and other researchers say, hypnotherapy potentially operates by modifying our state of awareness.

Imagine biting the nails, just trying to get rid of this poor habit. Timetable a consultation with a therapist to that end. The hypnotizer invites you to pick a position to rest, or even lay down when you reach the room. You are seated in a seat, and the hypnotherapist tells you what you intend to be focused on. You inform him that you want to quit chewing your fingers, so the therapist tells you to shut your eyes and pretend you're at your dream place, either on the shore or in a field. The hypnotherapist directs you via different images designed to help you feel at ease and peaceful. The hypnotherapist says if you're confident, you don't need to chew the nails anymore. He wants you to imagine clean, perfectly cut, un-bitten toes. This idea has a much more potent impact on the subconscious in your incredibly stable condition than it would otherwise have. Your extremely relaxed and confident emotional condition makes you extremely impressionable.

After you create the desired visual images, the hypnotist utilizes an expression like 'it's time to return to the moment' to persuade you to raise your eyes; the experience concludes with this.

The predominant hypnosis school of thought is that it is a manner of directly accessing an individual's subconscious mind. Usually, in the waking mind, you're still mindful of the thinking processes. You are actively talking about the challenges just next to you, intentionally using terms as you talk, actively trying to recall where you put the keys.

Yet in doing both of these things, the aware mind operates hand and glove with the subconscious mind, the involuntary portion of the mind that is concerned about your "behind the scenes." The subconscious mind uses the enormous data reservoir that allows you to fix issues, build paragraphs, or identify one's keys. It puts the ideas and plans together and runs them through the conscious mind. If a fresh concept appears out from the air to you, it's just that you have actually inadvertently gone about the system.

Even the subconscious takes control of all the things that you do unconsciously. You don't function consciously on the moment to moment relaxation procedures — that's what the subconscious manages. You don't go about any single thing you do when driving a vehicle-in your sub-consciousness, a lot of the little items are figured out. The bodily data your body gets too is processed by the subconscious.

In short, the mastermind behind the activity is the subconscious mind — it does all of your thinking, and it gets to decide a lot about what you are doing. Your thinking mind functions whilst you're still awake to analyze a number of such emotions, create choices, and bring those things into motion. It also stores and relays fresh knowledge to the subconscious. Yet while you're unconscious, the thinking mind stays out of path into the full rein of the subconscious.

Mental health professionals hypothesize that perhaps the hypnosis's intense relaxing and concentration techniques function to ease and disarm the cognitive mind until it plays a much less involved role in the thought cycle. You also are aware as to what is going on with this environment, but the rational brain comes second to the sub-consciousness. This helps one as well as the hypnotherapist to interact with the unconscious explicitly, efficiently. It is as if the cycle of hypnotism was opening up a settings menu within the head.

The two pieces of your mind control your life: your aware mind, and your subconscious mind. In general words, our thoughts "exist" in the sub-consciousness, and the rational brain defends and tries to justify them. The aware mind is the mind that "thinks," and the unconscious mind is really the mind that "feels." Self-control involves thought and originates in rational awareness. The trouble with this is that real, permanent improvement will only exist at the deep level of the emotion.

As progress occurs at just the underlying stage, it happens spontaneously and effortlessly, removing the stress and concentration needed while "attempting" and "having difficulties" with actively concentrated energy. Hypnosis helps one to "redo" the basic "scripts"-the thoughts, expectations, and perceptions we hold towards us in order to positively influence the conditioning inside ourselves and accomplish our goals.

You'll want to consume the food as you say to the self, "Do not eat wheat!" You give in to the bread before you realize it, and you speak to yourself in a bad way, and you don't have the courage to tell "NO." "Not allowing yourself only tends to lead to an "inevitable elephant kind of thought process," which

doesn't get you all that much closer to winning your goals in the longer run.

Rather what has to occur is that at the innate, "genuinely feel" stage, fresh, positive behaviors have to be developed by shifting attitudes, principles, and aspirations. This tends to happen by enhancing the capacity to spot bad feelings, feelings, or thinking even before it inevitably happens. It is here that the influence of hypnotherapy steps in.

Hypnotherapy operates by pressing into your unconscious mind's power and guiding that power toward your goals. Hypnosis is a normal state of concentrated concentration that enables one to obtain exposure to the dark, hidden part of you, the deeper level. Assume the sub-consciousness as a potent, motivated part within oneself that, if receive the proper instructions and encouragement, would then achieve its objectives you established for self. Envision your unconscious here as Geo-location that can support you does it point by point whether you have the right "target." Joining forces with the sub-consciousness allows one to optimize our full ability and to operate at a greater degree than simply involving the conscious mind. A qualified therapist or psychotherapist triggers a state of concentration and focus or

concentrated attention during the hypnosis. It is a method steered by linguistic signs and reiteration.

In so many respects, the dream-like state that people access may seem comparable to sleep, but you are completely aware of the situation. Your psychiatrist will make direct recommendations to help you reach your therapy objectives when you are in the hypnotic trance-like condition. Since you're in an elevated concentration, you might be quite open to new ideas or recommendations that you may neglect or shrug off in your usual mental state. The instructor will wake you up from the trance state when the process is done; otherwise, you will leave it yourself. It's uncertain if the effect this extreme degree of internal commitment and centered awareness is having. Throughout the trance-like state, hypnosis may position the seedlings of different motivations in your mind, and soon those processes take origin and flourish. In addition, hypnosis can clear a path for stronger processes and recognition. If it's "cluttered" in your regular mental state, your mind might not be capable of absorbing suggestions and guidance.

Here's a fast way to explain hypnotherapy: hypnosis is an extremely calm emotional condition in which the conscious mind is bypassed. That is to say; the brain is calm and eager to follow; the spirit is even more open to advice.

We will bypass certain unconscious thoughts in thoroughly relaxing hypnotherapy, and refresh this reasoning with fresh ideas. Hypnosis operates by encouraging us to change our internal mechanisms of thought to help us attain particular goals.

Here's an example: Assume you need to use hypnotherapy to lose weight.

The inner self retains other assumptions in weight management. You may think instantly: It's hard to lose weight, you do not want to abandon your favorite foods, or you don't have enough time for the gym. Ultimately, these mental processes – shaped by recollections, perspectives, and expectations – drive our conscious behavior, and we don't even recognize it is happening.

In essence, the unconscious mind is setting us up for disappointment. And that's true of so many of our unhealthy habits — poor self-talk, cigarettes, binge eating — all of which are firmly rooted in the subconscious thinking.

However, by hypnotherapy, we will start modifying and reviewing these harmful beliefs. And this may clarify why the

evidence clearly indicates this hypnosis operates with problems such as debilitating pain, misuse of drugs, and calorie restriction.

By teaching our psyches to think about problems and aspirations differently, we will eradicate the anxious feelings, which too often contribute to self-sabotage.

Hypnotherapy just said enables you to modify one's automatic mind. And this is the way hypnotherapy functions, in summary.

Our brains have repetitive habits profoundly rooted. So these habits of thinking evolve during a lifespan. Recollections, theories, negative feelings, optimistic encounters-all help shape and strengthen certain habits and convictions.

To put it one way, everything we experience, smell, perceive, and believe is real is not necessarily right. Rather, our cognitive perceptions – which we assume to be real – are formed by evolving brain networks that process sensory evidence.

This is regarded as a top-down delivery. In top-down management, the knowledge that comes from the surface supersedes and tells processes at the lower stage.

Here's an instance: Assume you're staring at a red vehicle. Visibly the eye catches the car's visual cues. Such information is forwarded to advanced tiers of neural synapses in which the form and color are decrypted. Then, this knowledge moves to higher stages of processing, where color and design enable us to distinguish the build and model of the vehicle.

The information radiates outward, but the sum of input moves down around 10 times at the very exact time. This top-down feedback determined by the unconscious thoughts tells the brain how sensory data can be interpreted. Here is an explanation of how hypnotherapy succeeds. Through fresh, more constructive ideas to circumvent the top-down systems, participants are willing to view the environment from different eyes.

Only consider the Stroop effect. When staring at the term Blue, it is hard to tell "color," since our minds interpret the term blue immediately until we decipher the hue of the dye. But in perceiving the terms as gibberish, we may skip the skeptical and address the query without hesitation.

That's the secret to getting past poor behaviors and self-improvement. We have to get to the underlying cause-our pessimistic expectations that hold the terrible habit in place-

and replace them with stronger, more beneficial details. Then you will transcend the experienced top-down mechanisms in your brain – that is, when you experience pain, you desire sugar – and substitute this thought with a more constructive approach.

Re-wiring our predisposed convictions by hypnotherapy is a powerful method for change. The strength of the predisposed convictions is a perfect illustration here. A group of participants was asked to take a taste check of the wine. Two options were offered to them: a glass of "cheap" wine, and another of reasonably priced wine.

The reality was: All containers had similar champagne. And yet participants expected the costly bottle to taste better, and thus gave it much higher taste marks. The proposal was nuanced; one was more costly-but it shows clearly how quickly an idea can be used to build our belief. The logical brain is sad, not that open to suggestion. You listen to an idea, after which you evaluate it, and you criticize it. But with hypnosis, we allow the mind to consider ideas better? Our brains become more sensitive about advice in the profoundly calm condition of hypnosis.

Thanks to two concepts, people are able to re-frame their thought patterns: Suggestion and disassociation.

- **Disassociation**: When in a condition of hypnotherapy, the idea is that the consciousness splits into two bodies – the mesmerized subconscious and the listener concealed. In other terms, we should blank out our environment and circumvent current top-down thought (the outsider hidden). This enables us to accept recommendations without worrying about how the idea applies to our personal thoughts. And new work into brain scans shows that hypnotherapy may establish brain associations that will solve this issue.

- **Suggestion**: The mesmerized individual is guided to concentrate on a particular thought, or recommendation, throughout hypnosis. And when you have entered the mesmerized zone, you will override the rational thought on the recommendations. That's one hypothesis about how hypnotherapy operates; we arrive at a condition where the subconscious can create ideas without challenging them. Only look at the experiment of Dr. Raz: The mesmerized participants interpret easily familiar terms as word salad – BLUE, White, etc. That was when the subconscious was able to function on advice without knowing why.

In the end, sensory input suits our top-down thinking much of the time. We see a red car, and our recollections tell us how to perceive and decrypt what the car is. But, by developing a discrepancy among bottom-up and top-down thinking, hypnosis is working.

Using hypnosis, we utilize advice to teach the mind to react differently – to construct a new environment in which sensory input causes better, more productive responses. Therefore, whenever you encounter discomfort, your current top-down thoughts can encourage you to try to reach for a regular cigarette, or snack on sugary snacks, or remain up at night – hypnosis helps one to refresh and re-frame all these top-down responses.

Our preconditioned conviction shapes truth. We hope to like a nice bottle of wine differently as it's more costly; we experience a disparity in like. Our minds view terms as nonsensical gibberish, and we will, without hesitation, discern the hue of the paper. Hypnosis offers the ability to overcome our current convictions, hypotheses, and experiences. This is accomplished by pursuing an entrancing initiation, where we enter a trance.

When we enter hypnosis, we are better able to dissociate our mental stimuli and rational thinking as per the state principle of hypnosis. In several other terms, we should receive and obey advice while asking whether we are doing those. In the final analysis, it is the force of persuasion that helps one to re-define and re-frame our experiences.

To put it another way, our minds have a dynamic network to view the environment surrounding. With time, involuntary pessimistic and counterproductive emotions made their way through the web. Thus people feel a huge desire to consume in candy, or smoke cigarettes, or take to illegal substances when humans feel anxiety. Unrestricted are such latent impulses. They eventually occur.

Yet hypnotherapy helps one to conquer such wild emotions and to lessen them. And this is where the strength lies: Hypnotherapy allows us to accept ideas that suit us the most to be real. That, in fact, helps us to improve our actions.

Hypnosis and Brain Waves

The brain is always busy. Right now, it's full to the brim with beta waves when you read the document. When your mind wanders, maybe more alpha waves would be created when you drift off and start fantasizing. And if you totally nod off, you can record a higher percentage of delta waves. Wherever you may be or what you do, there is always a certain brain - wave process like this is happening. Your incredible brain

comprises trillions of neuron cells.

Such neurons interact with one another through electric charges. The waves may be quantified utilizing a Brainwave device, an EEG, while they are interacting. So such messages can manifest as various forms of brainwaves based on what you're doing at the moment. Brainwaves, or Hertz, are quantified in cycles/ second. They have a speed calculated in times per second; that is their pace. We do have intensity, which is the real wave scale or height. In some brain regions, the higher the speed, the more phases per second (hertz), so the more brain function there is.

Knowing what happens during hypnotherapy or self-hypnosis will help to explain how and why it functions. The various variations in brainwave rhythms each offer their own advantages.

You may conceive of brainwaves as radio waves that have a number of various speeds/ frequency range, each with its own features. They are all present along a spectrum, with one predominating condition. When you read this, there is indeed a strong probability that you will be mostly in Beta, which is our normal style of fasting. Ideally, wide open, ready, and diligent!

If we shut our eyes, we will calm and concentrate on sleep, contemplation, yoga, or hypnosis in the slower spectrum of Alpha brainwave. Calm, awake, aware, and confident; we can be comfortable here.

The next region down in the spectrum is much slower, darker, and more reserved as the waves of Theta predominate. This is the central rhythm of brainwave, as we go to bed or dream. Even so, you remain alert in hypnosis while you can feel incredibly comfortable. Delta is the weakest deepest waves, but these are achieved in very deep slumber or in the strongest meditation.

The zones that we want to reach in hypnosis are the Alpha and Theta brainwaves in hypnotherapy or self-hypnosis as you start to unwind and be more self-focused, and move into patterns of alpha waves. This helps you to enter the region where memory retention is theoretically enhanced, reduced discomfort, reduced levels of anxiety, and a smoother reaction to stress.

As the trance-like condition intensifies, we will only control the vibrations of the Theta. There we are in a context where we are growing our internal knowledge. We should be completely confident, relying on the feedback from inside and providing learning and improving space. There is another important aspect of these two brain wave zones besides obtaining these vibrational states and their corresponding characteristics and advantages. We're more open to ideas in both the Alpha and Theta states. We can start exploring new and meaningful ways to work with unconstructive lifestyles or old values and beliefs, using this responsive state.

The concept of having affirmations is also familiar to individuals, and they may be very beneficial. When you use hypnosis or self-hypnosis to work with this idea, you have the chance to make them deeper, so they can become "turbo-charged" statements.

Everything humans think has an effect on their attitudes and, therefore, can affect their biology. When we dream about or witness anything upsetting, then we get the symptoms of tension. These symptoms can be rage, anger, fear, depression, etc., and the autonomic reaction (cortisol and adrenaline) that produces a reaction like a fight, freeze. Such reactions are brilliant in a completely life-threatening circumstance but not for our safety in the long run.

Using a method to moving your brain activity rhythms to a more comfortable state will give you a micro-holiday from everyday life's pressures and strains. You will shift the perspective by building an inner refuge at that moment and enabling calm feelings to circulate and getting more confident in enjoying the advantages of the body. Then you can nurture yourself in your alpha and theta states by relying on constructive thoughts, pictures, and concepts, dealing through challenges and barriers to starting opening possibilities.

When you get entranced, there are various stages that you go to. Every now and again, some people really can't wrap their heads around the idea that they can hear, recall, and understand any or all of what the hypnotherapist says during the hypnotherapy sessions.

Your brain can supply a variety of waves, but they generally fall through one of the four kinds mentioned below.

- **Beta Waves**

They're waves with elevated frequency, low intensity. In basic words, when you are thinking, when you're alert, you emit beta waves. Such waves are correlated with anything you perform in a waking mind, like Reading Rational Thought Sleeping Dining Communicating Walking Problem Solving Any time you concentrate on it, there are more beta waves. When you actively tap into your memory reserves, they are triggered too. The aspect to note here is that such waves aren't mutually exclusive. During every particular moment, they are all active in the brain. So you'll have greater beta wave action than any of the other three forms while you're up, finding out the solution to a question, reading a book or a webpage, or engaged in discussion with a buddy. But there are also some other forms, perhaps not as strong.

This level of consciousness can be calculated by frequency (Hz) using an electroencephalograph. It can be defined as a conscious awakening. You are aware, fully awake, and you can hear, understand, and fully comprehend it all when you communicate with the therapist. Your aware vital mind is triggered during this time, and you react to preconceived beliefs in your psyche, acting on such beliefs on a day-to-day basis.

When you're engaging in behavioral tasks, the prevailing brainwave status is Beta, so it's normal for people to spend much of the working day generating Beta brainwaves. Neurons pulse quickly through the brain in the Beta state, leading to optimum results. Athletes, chief leaders, strong politicians, and highly experienced students emit Beta brainwaves while working to their full ability. The beta brainwave states lead to frequencies between 12 Hz and 40

Hz. People can choose any Beta brainwave template audios if they are involved in growing their focus, motivation, and profitability.

- **Alpha Waves**

Alpha waves arise throughout relaxed and comfortable phases, taking up the spectrum around 8 and 12 Hz. Although beta waves reflect your state of consciousness, alpha waves serve as a link among the conscious and the unconscious. When the nervous system is at rest, more alpha-waves are generated. Alpha waves activate in the brain when the thought processes float the brain. You are quiet though not completely breathing deeply. The alpha state is sometimes defined as being in the "now" or present-day here. These vibrations are weaker than those of Beta, so Alpha is good for studying. It allows one the room and quietness of mind to consume and absorb knowledge. And shutting your eyes immediately helps the brain emit more alpha waves. Also, the alpha state is helpful for concentrated meditation, reduced stress, and fear, and helped manage discomfort.

You are relaxed, and your brainwave level decreases, as you start listening to the voice in the bed. The reticular activation system in your brain is beginning to slow down and take a little hiatus from your conscious mind. Ultimately you fall to Alpha, which is estimated at 7.5-14Hz. You will hear and comprehend the therapist throughout this process. You can proceed with any directed simulation that he or she suggests; use your creativity in a vibrant way. Throughout this process, your brain is really open to the ideas that are offered to you.

Alpha brainwaves are often slower than Beta brainwaves and arise during sleep, meditation, and imagination. The state of Alpha is an incredibly satisfying, healthy state of mind. Alpha brainwaves are connected to profound degrees of imagination, understanding, and motivation. Artists, singers, and performers produce an excess of alpha brainwaves, consistent with high output. Alpha brainwaves are important in raising amounts of cortisol, raising the negative consequences of stress, and strengthening the immune system. The brainwave alpha states lead to wavelengths varying from 8 Hz to 12 Hz. You can choose one of the Alpha brainwave pattern audios if you are trying to improve imagination, reach optimum output and foster a state of calm consciousness.

What scientists equate with "right-brain" operation, or our collective senses of thought, ingenuity, memory, and insight, is an "alpha state of mind." You're supposed to be in an alpha condition while the brain wave output falls down to around 8 and 12 Hz. It's called a "comfortable" state of mind that encourages you to be more sensitive, more accessible, more imaginative, and less critical. Edison, Einstein, and several other great minds found their research to be a regular process of reaching an alpha-state of mind. We have stronger memory recall when using alpha state. And since we're relaxed, we seem to be more concentrated, making smarter choices.

In sleep, while daydreaming, or more deliberately with Mindfulness and Self Hypnosis, we connect this state quite rapidly. In fact, your brain will plunge into an alpha state numerous times during the day, even when you're waking with your eyes wide open. Learning to reach an alpha state will benefit you to improve memory, imagination, and insight, so if you are trained daily — just for brief times — you will be able to improve tension more quickly, and your stress will decrease.

One might ask, "How to move into an Alpha State of mind?" The Silva Meditation Methods provide the simplest, most effective approach to achieve the alpha state easily and consistently for over twenty years now. You may also use some activation for self-hypnosis, or any mediation entry form to move into an alpha condition. Or you can only keep your eyes closed and start counting 100 to 1, reminding one that you are moving further. All types of self-induced change of mind normally involve some type of self-hypnosis or auto-suggestion. It simply means that we start taking direct control of our state of mind and are able to create the change internally by using affirmation or mental visualization.

- **Theta Waves**

The aware brain is in control while you're awake. There are Beta waves in motion. Alpha waves are becoming more prominent as you continue to get more comfortable. You're nevertheless fully conscious but really laid back. Theta waves then pick up the slack when your unconscious mind takes over. Such vibrations are in the range of 4 to 8 Hertz. Naturally, you can create more theta waves while you are: Intensely calm Practice Daydreaming Vision In a deep trance state Approaching Sleep These waves are weaker again, placing you right on the brink of sleep. They are often defined as sleeping in stage 1, and being in the dusk state. You will feel it as you lie in bed, right before you fall asleep. You know you are lying in bed, even if you lack the feeling of lying in bed. And if in this condition you don't fall asleep, such pretty stunning stuff will happen. Your thinking mind is almost turned off when theta frequencies are powerful.

That implies you can unlock your implicit potentials. You should join in with the imaginative side. You should settle for your instincts. You will think about intense sleep, and feel it. People can dig deep within and start calling recollections. Theta waves are connected to memory, the emotion it's something called "neuroplasticity," which means your brain can reorganizeitself in the theta state. For starters, when you discover anything new, the brain requires time to take in it. It will have to both transcribe and store the information for later. This is done by creating new relationships among neurons. Any of these different interactions are altering the brain ever so slightly. So this is one of the factors we use hypnosis, as it helps you to create permanent brain improvements.

As you begin to relax, the amplitude of the brainwave can fall deeper downward to Theta. Stuff at this stage may start feeling a little blurry. During this time, your mind may wander away, and you may even lose parts of what the therapist says. This is completely normal, and it implies that your subconscious mind listens to suggestions and acts accordingly.

- **Delta Waves**

Delta waves happen while you're dreaming. These are just the weakest frequency bands that you can generate, which occupy the lower end of the spectrum up to 4 Hz. The longer you rest, the greater the intensity of delta waves. But even if you're resting, it doesn't imply there's not anything going on here. Delta waves are especially effective in helping you: get a good night's sleep. Promoting healing from the inside out naturally enhances your immune system. The aged you get less and fewer delta waves you generate. This helps me understand the term "sleep like an infant." Delta waves are often necessary to control all of your involuntary biological functions, like the pulse rate and metabolism. Delta is the highest hypnosis condition. Delta is a profoundly curative condition, and you are not sure of what the therapist is doing at the period, but the ideas are acknowledged.

You will remember that in your hypnotherapy session, it is uncommon for you to reach only one condition. More possibly, you may start by fluctuating between Alphas to Theta, and often you may fall down to Delta as you are more acquainted with the therapist's speech. Many clients say that they believe they've gone to sleep as they respond to hypnotherapy MP3s, but when the recording ends, they reopen their eyeballs. This is one illustration of Delta.

As you can see, when you get hypnotized, there are multiple forms you could go through each of these stages is equally successful. And if you're concerned that it didn't succeed during your first experience of hypnosis, take consolation in the knowledge that you just need to be in a really mild condition (Alpha) to be successful with the treatment.

Theta brainwaves are much higher in duration and arise through intense stages of relaxing, sleep, hypnosis, and enhanced imagination. In the change from alertness to sleeping and even while dreaming, they also are noticed. Spending extended quantities of the period in a Theta condition will greatly boost the physical well-being and well-being, resulting in decreased sleeping needs. In the Theta state, the consciousness is in harmony with the heart of the earth's vibrational force. You can quickly reach the inner force in the Theta Zone, and achieve higher degrees of consciousness. The Theta condition is the brain wave model that many hypnotists utilize on their patients while performing behavioral hypnosis, as the subconscious is more responsive to entrancing stimuli when in the Theta condition. Theta brainwave rhythms vary from 4 Hz to 8Hz in frequencies. You can choose any of the Theta brainwave template audios if you are trying to gain from hypnotic feedback and reach deep degrees of relaxation synonymous with harmony and tranquility.

Delta brainwave patterns are the slowest of the wavelengths of the brainwave, which are detected during intense, dreamless sleep, while they can often be experienced in deep meditation. Delta waves are correlated with intense relaxation rates, optimum physical regeneration, and the aging cycle slowing down. Delta brainwaves refer to the 0 Hz to 4 Hz ranges. You can choose any of the Delta brainwave rhythm audios if you are trying to attain warm, restorative sleep, and the highest degree of relaxation correlated with physical recovery and halting the aging cycle.

Auto-suggestions

Some hypnotism is founded upon auto-suggestion. A "self-recommendation" or "self-suggestion" is a recommendation you are offering to yourself. It can take the shape of visual confirmation or a mental picture at times. In the early 1840s, the Scottish psychiatrist and physician, James Braid, the father of hypnotherapy, discovered self-hypnosis. Braid did not use the term "auto-suggestion," but he described hypnotherapy as an "expectant, prevailing thought" condition of focused attention. Therefore Braid assumed that all the hypnosis was basically self-hypnosis. He later likened, as he simply named it, "self-hypnotism" to the trance methods of old Hindu yoga, while maintaining that hypnotism operated by clear, rational thinking, psychological concepts.

Do not use verbal derogatory words such as "less nervous," "not biting my lip," "not upset," etc. Sigmund Freud once wrote, 'There are no negation, no uncertainty, and no degree of confidence in this method. There is the only material in the unconscious, invested with greater or lesser energy.'

The explanation of the stereotypes is: "Don't think about blue horses. You may think about any creature you like but not blue horses." To grasp the significance of those terms, most individuals do want to talk of horses specifically! Simply placed, this occurs randomly at the edge of your consciousness in order to grasp a term you normally have to elicit any memory or emotion from your context that gives it significance. You'll picture the terms material, irrespective of the sentence's context. Therefore, "I feel less nervous" is a weak idea that is more effective than suppressing negative feelings. "I feel more at ease" is even easier as it allows you to focus on what trust entails. Say the auto-suggestions favorably, and say what you want, not something you don't want.

Use the current tense is typically easier than utilizing past or hypothetical forms. "I'm getting calmer" or "I'm relaxed and optimistic" is easier than "I'm going to be cool." Future ideas may be included, but they're best related to actual circumstances and worded in the present continuous. "I'm relaxed and comfortable when I rise to deliver my speech at the wedding," for example, is stronger than "I'm going to be cool at the wedding." Phrasing it in the present tense promotes connection with the moment, and is more apt to elicit an emotional or physical reaction than utilizing the past or potential tense, and induces a sense of isolation and dissociation.

The word auto-suggestion refers to all ideas, and then all self-administered sensations that enter one's mind across the five senses. The auto-suggestion is self-suggestion, to put it another way. It is the coordination agent between that portion of the mind where rational thinking occurs, and that which represents the subconscious mind as the seat of operation.

1.4 Deep Sleep Hypnosis for Insomnia

Sleep hypnosis includes responding to auditory suggestions by a therapist that is meant through the force of persuasion to bring one into a trance-like condition. Hypnotists use multiple methods to promote sleep, such as intense focus, control of the symptoms, and guided imaging. A person who is now being entranced can hear phrases like "relax," "quiet," "easy," and "let go." Such terms are intended to persuade someone to sleep away.

Hypnosis is a nap-like, or trance-like, a mental state in which the mind is entirely relaxed and open to some suggestions from outside. In order to achieve this state securely and effectively, a qualified therapist is usually required.

Sleep hypnosis is often used to make people fall asleep, remain asleep, and have healthier sleep hours. A person listens to signs prompting relaxation response and stimulates a state in which drifting off to sleep is easier.

Sleep hypnosis may be done with a tape or by a therapist. It can be a collection of repetitive terms as you reflect on what and little that is being mentioned. It can be soothing music with visual driven tips placing you in the perfect atmosphere for relaxing and deep sleep.

You are completely in charge of your mind and spirit, contrary to certain old values.

Sleep hypnosis is a session where a hypnotist directs a client through verbal inputs that induce relaxation, in person or via an audio, and a trance-like session that can be used to help you sleep drift. Hypnotist helps the subject to actively "sleep," while still unconsciously alert. The consequent trance-like state takes place with low-level brainwave activity, i.e., the Delta, Theta, alpha states where rational activity wanes, and subconscious activity increases. You should also use sleep hypnotherapy to bring the patient into a relaxing and rehabilitative state.

A sleep hypnosis session typically includes:

- **Getting relaxed**: The recipient settles down and becomes comfortable.

- **Letting go**: The participant is directed to set away from any fears or doubts.

- **The induction**: This gets ready for the participant to go deeper into relaxation through releasing the rational mind and going to open up the subconscious.

- **Relaxation**: This segment involves deliberate relaxation that makes the user relax evermore.

- **The suggestions**: This is the lengthiest and final part of the hypnosis, directed visualization that plants the intended outcome into the subconscious mind of the participant.

Sleep hypnotherapy is an effective and safe way if done properly, to drift off to slumber. It is believed a patient must be transparent and trust in the concept of sleep therapy to be successful.

You should offer sleep hypnosis a shot and see how it will help you sleep peacefully before heading for the sleeping tablets. Sleep hypnosis can be applied to the sleep routine as a discipline, along with certain routines that you implement.

If you've done certain things like creating a comfortable, quiet, and dark environment to fall asleep and still experience insomnia, perhaps it's time to try hypnosis for sleeping. Most people report that due to sleep hypnosis, they sleep easier and even deeper.

You go through phases as you sleep. The first two stages are where dreaming will be heard. With the REM (Rapid Eye Movement) providing the deepest stage of sleep, the last two cycles are considered as deep sleep. These periods are without visions. These periods are the most essential because they are the most restorative. Over the night, you go through these loops many times. Studies indicate that

How Does It Work?

You lie in bed, and you battle your mind. You talk about the almost endless to-do checklist for tomorrow. Your body aspires to sleep. Yet you do have other things on your head.

Chances are you've had that in your life. 50 to 70 million Americans struggle from a sleeping or alertness condition according to research. And that may illustrate why we're only averaging 6.8 hours sleep a night.

In other terms, we are deprived of regular sleep, and this sleep deprivation reduces the ability of the human body to properly rejuvenate, heal, and recover itself. Yet insomnia sleep hypnosis may provide a cure, allowing us to get to sleep more easily. Sleep is the key to well-being.

Our cells regenerate themselves, naturally, all through sleep. Hormone rates are being balanced, the subconscious is being renewed, and a number of critical health mechanisms are taking place. In short, we're placing our emotional and physical well-being at risk while we deny ourselves of adequate sleep. Sadly it's not always easy to reset the body rhythm to accomplish deep, restful shut-eye.

In short, our subconscious minds hide multiple sleep disturbances deep inside. At bedtime, discomfort exceeds thoughts of sleepiness. We let anxiety taint our thoughts, and as a consequence, we simply cannot seem to be able to silence our inner scripts and get to sleep.

Yet insomnia hypnosis provides a cure. Sleep hypnotherapy

includes a path chart to plan, calm, and encourage sleep. In addition, hypnosis will help us resolve tiredness in bedtime, unwind faster, and finally collapse into a warm, restful sleep.

In basic words, the hypnosis of sleep or insomnia is a method used to trigger deep sleep, which is close to conventional hypnosis. You take measures at bedtime to attain physically and mentally calm, and if you enter this comfortable and concentrated condition, you can provide feedback that will help the body fall into relaxation.

Hypnosis is a coma-like mental state in which the entranced person practices profound relaxation, concentrated attention, and higher open-mindedness to a recommendation. Hypnosis is believed to be a way of gaining better access to the unconscious mind of the individual and, at the same time, diminishing the possibility that the participant will infuse aware worries, anxiety, or reallocation into the treatment process.

Hypnosis is commonly used to change habits and responses that may lead to underlying health issues (like insomnia and other sleep disturbances), owing to its potential to improve sensitivity. Your battle to sleep may be fueled by multiple factors.

Anxiety and stress, for example, — two of the major contributors — affect your ability to "shut off" your mind before bed. Even medical conditions such as asthma or allergies may keep you awake. Or the trigger may be anything as apparently insignificant as a daily shift.

However, we're kept alive in several situations by our inner conversations. And thus will assist with anxiety hypnotherapy.

The mind could be running, worrying about a traumatic situation coming up (like the first week of a job.) Or you could constantly revisit unanswered issues from the day on in your head. Sleep hypnotherapy for insomnia provides a mechanism for helping our minds to turn off, allowing our body to reach a calm state, and eventually pushing us from hypnotic sleep trance. A sleep-promoting hypnotherapy regimen in particular benefits you to:

- **Calm You Physically**: hypnosis, in general, offers strategies for relieving body pain, calming muscles, and maintaining the sense of heaviness in the body. The body is completely relaxed under hypnosis, which can be accomplished by breathing and focusing techniques.

- **Relax Mentally**: The entrancing condition is a condition of heightened consciousness and concentration, almost like meditation. By pursuing the methods of hypnosis, you will start unburdening the brain of its anxiety. You desire to step on from your waking mind and to feel a separation from your world. As such, sleep hypnotherapy is beneficial as it lets you slow down your inner feelings, block them out, or concentrate elsewhere.

- **Induce Relaxation**: In common belief, a hypnotic coma isn't meditation. You stay conscious and alert. The shift from a hypnosis state to sleep is instinctual, however. Both have parallels, and therefore, after you've psychologically and physically recovered, basic ideas will help you fall into sleep.

- **Falling into Deep Sleep**: Work has found that listening to a tape of sleep hypnosis before bed will help us get to deep slumber more easily. In reality, a study in 2014 showed that women who were listening to a recording of sleep hypnosis before bed lasted eight times longer in deep slumber. Hypnosis, in other words, helps us to drift off to sleep faster, remain asleep longer; helps ensure that we spend much time in the intended Rapid eye movement sleep stages.

Insomnia is one of the most popular sleep conditions, and the disease may have a significant effect on the quality of life for persistent sufferers. There are several common forms of insomnia.

Sleeplessness may be short-term. Of starters, a shift in schedule, a disorder, hormones, sadness, or fear will all make it hard to fall asleep. Luckily you adjust to a regular sleep pattern in just a few days or even weeks in most situations.

In comparison, long-term, recurrent insomnia applies to persistent and long-term sleep disruptions. If you have had difficulty sleeping for more than a couple of months three days a week, perhaps the insomnia is persistent.

Alternatively, insomnia can be called insomnia as "sleep onset" or insomnia as "sleep-maintenance." Sleep initiation relates to experiencing problems sleeping, whereas sleep management applies to problems sleeping. Hypnotherapy provides a means to mitigate the underlying cause of all kinds of insomnia.

Chronic insomniacs continue to have anxious over falling asleep; they train the mind to believe it would be a challenge to fall asleep. So it buries this learning deep inside the amygdala. Some individuals will begin to re-frame some implicit feelings by hypnosis and create more meaningful experiences. For example, a tape or hypnotherapist may use encouraging terms like "peace," "rest," or "quietness" to explain bedtime and sleep during a sleep hypnotherapy session. It aims to untangle the unconscious subconscious from harmful experiences.

Sleep hypnosis provides a step-by-step method for severe sufferers to clear waking emotions, achieve a condition of physical and emotional calm, and ready the body and mind for bed. Usually, acute insomnia is attributed to tension or anxiety. You are worried about the day, or you are nervous over things coming up. By utilizing hypnosis, you have a structure for the subconscious to shut down more efficiently.

1.5 Benefits Of Hypnosis

Hypnosis has many benefits due to its ability to surpass the logical mind. You become open when you're hypnotized in a way that enables you to overcome the restrictive biases and defensive systems that keep you abound, whenever your rational mind is at the forefront. Both body and mind you are absolutely comfortable. And at all stages, you remain in full possession of yourself and your senses, so you are not sleeping. It sounds like a lot of daydreaming or reflection, but most people find it relaxing and restorative. Hypnotherapy requires having a particular target, as does sleep, whereas daydreaming is usually more casual.

Hypnosis may be used to alter a wide variety of behaviors and traumatic perceptions, which we'll discuss in more detail below. It is widely used, for example, to improve self-esteem, losing weight, phobia, smoking abstinence, anxiety, and certain types of chronic pain.

In theory, however, hypnosis should be used to deal with just about any problem which has a neurological dimension and includes harmful ways of thought. When you stick to social progress, there is no end on what you will do.

Some people agree that one session is enough to make them relax or behave better whilst others prefer a longer hypnotherapy course. But, the usage of "top-up" sessions to hold successful progress is often popular—most people who use recordings for hypnotherapy show at least some progress within three weeks. Many continue with regular sessions, dwindling slowly to weekly or monthly.

Hypnosis is a technique founded on research that is well-supported as a therapy for a wide variety of unhealthy patterns of behavior. Studies, for example, suggest that hypnosis is successful in addressing the following:

Habits

As we replicate certain patterns, they get entrenched to create a set of stimuli that make us continue to reproduce certain habits. People who over-eat, for example, maybe doing so caused by pain, depression, and isolation. Hypnotherapy will help you identify and neutralize causes for over-eating, smoking, alcohol, compulsive gaming, and job avoidance.

Since hypnotizing allows you to be more suggestive than normal, there has been proof that it can help you quit unhealthy habits such as drinking or smoking.

Professionals explain that a session usually involves a hypnotist generating a bad connotation with the smoking experience, such as having a particularly dry throat after that, which will discourage the smoker next time. And if you have an addiction that you simply can't curb, that could be the key to hypnosis.

Thanks to routine and repetition, behaviors are profoundly rooted in our thought. There are several causes for smokers: heat, breakfast and dinner timings, driving, and frustration, to mention only a handful. Hypnosis helps individuals to analyze and relieve themselves of these involuntary stimuli. Smoking, drug misuse, drinking, binge eating, and laziness

may improve in hypnosis.

Phobias

Once you formed a crippling fear early on in life, it may be particularly difficult to recall its roots or to get rid of the anxiety. These contradictory ideas and perceptions may be deconstructed and modified by hypnosis. As starters, whether you're terrified of flight, actual surgical treatments, interpersonal interaction, or social speaking, hypnosis will help you get past such phobias. Anxiety: whether you're too nervous (whether about different issues or general), hypnosis will even help you cultivate a more positive outlook about the personal causes. Anxiety also keeps people from taking reasonable chances, and approaching them in this manner will help you make strides in your professional growth.

Medical Conditions

Every medical disorder that includes a mental aspect is a subject for hypnosis help. Hypnosis, for instance, will enable you to reform the biases and fears that build a stressful loop surrounding sleep, whether you have trouble sleeping. Other disorders, reproductive disorders, and symptoms of health anxiety can be likewise enhanced. Hypnosis may even change the unconscious mechanisms that trigger the teeth to grit in

bruxism at night). Other disorders, emotional disorders, and symptoms of health anxiety can be likewise enhanced.

Scientific Research trials have strongly confirmed the efficacy of the hypnosis on IBS. IBS is the bowel-created stomach discomfort, so hypnotherapy may also relieve signs like indigestion, vomiting so heartburn.

IBS may also induce effects such as diarrhea, exhaustion, back pain, and bladder issues. Hypnosis has proven that it can assist with those symptoms too. Hypnosis takes you into gradual healing, offering calming thoughts and stimuli to combat the symptoms.

Sleep

You enter a sleep-like condition, but stay alert while you perform hypnosis. Seeing how similar it is to dreaming through hypnotherapy, it is simple to see how insomnia will benefit you and encourage healthier sleep.

According to the professionals, hypnotic advice should be used to prepare the subconscious to establish more restful night-time habits. Hypnosis may be a valuable method if you are sleepwalking or unable to fall and remain asleep. Hypnosis will calm you enough just to help you to sleep easier if you do have sleeplessness. Hypnosis will also teach you to stay in bed whenever you sense your feet touch the floor to help you stop sleepwalking misadventures if you're a sleepwalker. And if you only want to have a little more night, hypnosis will even assist with that. Using the methods of self-hypnosis will improve the length of time you rest and the length of time you spend in deep slumber — the sort of rest you have to have to wake up to feel renewed.

How it works is that verbal signals place you in a trance-like environment, close to how you experience when you're so absorbed in a book or video that you don't realize what's happening around you. You'll fall asleep during hypnosis or just after that.

Anxiety and Depression

If you get lots of anxiety (whether about particular issues or general), hypnotherapy will often help you build a more positive outlook toward the personal stimuli, anxiety also keeps people from undertaking reasonable chances, and approaching them in this manner will help you make strides in your professional growth.

Stress Hypnosis, which involves those diagnosed with depression or anxiety, may help change the thinking processes.

Individuals with depression or anxiety have recorded successful effects by being handled with hypnotherapy as an alternate treatment.

Tension is no fun to contend with, which is why hypnotherapy is listed by the Wellness Institute as an effective remedy for stress and anxiety.

For someone who is not involved in taking drugs but who needs to re-wire unhealthy behavioral patterns like cyclical thought or obsessed, it is a nice idea to try. Hypnosis will help you change your reasoning process and develop a more positive mindset.

Adaptive hypnotherapy incorporating hypnosis and psycho-behavioral treatment, when communicating with the subconscious, aims to alter unhealthy habits and behaviors. Experts claim this therapy will relieve the "jammed" habits of behavior that cause stress, stress, Obsessive-compulsive disorder as well as other mental illnesses.

Worries are always unfounded and will mess with the way of life. Hypnotherapy allows us to explore our problems and offer fresh insights that will help us create more meaningful connections. Hypnosis can assist with: general fear, social anxiety, anxiety for tests, situation panic, anxiety for success, and public speaking.

Stress reduction methods — hypnosis involved — will also relieve fear. Hypnosis appears to be most successful in patients whose distress is triggered by a specific disorder of well-being — like a cardiac failure — instead of by a general fear.

Hypnosis will also benefit if you are dealing with an irrational fear — a form of stress condition when you become deeply scared of anything which doesn't present a major threat.

How it helps: Hypnotherapy helps to relieve fear by stimulating the body to trigger its normal reaction to stimulation through utilizing an expression or non-verbal signal, slowing down breathing, reducing heart rate, and inculcating an immediate sense of vitality.

Pain Management

Any kind of pain, let alone severe pain, is not good. Those experiencing persistent pain may consider seeking extreme measures to treat it, although it does not have to be so severe at all. Work has shown that hypnotherapy can help relieve and alleviate persistent pain. Because most pain is simply caused by the brain, it makes sense that a psychiatric treatment such as hypnosis may be effective in controlling

pain.

Hypnosis was used to relieve all common pain forms (neuropathy, fibromyalgia, ulcerative colitis), and severe injury pain. A research released in the Global Publication of Medical and Behavioral Hypnotism showed that hypnotherapy utilizing augmented reality technologies decreased pain severity greater than traditional care alone in admitted critically ill patients.

Hypnosis may assist relieve pain — such as during surgery, migraines, or hallucinations with stress. Also, persistent pain can improve, too. People with pain associated with conditions such as inflammation, chemotherapy, sickle cell anemia, and fibromyalgia — as well as those with lower back pain — can feel hypnosis relief.

How it works: Hypnosis will allow you to deal with pain and develop better self-control over pain. However, findings show that hypnotherapy over extended stretches of time will achieve so successfully.

Weight Loss

Shape Magazine states that hypnosis is not a cure for a diet, but instead a means to resolve emotional obstacles that hinder weight reduction, such as excessive eating or avoidance of exercise.

If hypnotism is also used in conjunction with improvements in nutrition and activity, it is typically most effective. How it works is very interesting. When you're hypnotized, the emphasis is on the mind. It helps you most likely to react and adapt to ideas about improvements in your lifestyle, such as following a healthier lifestyle or exercising regularly, which may keep you healthy.

Low self-esteem

Low self-esteem people usually have a very strong "mental critic "— a voice that suggests they're not smart enough, that they're doomed to struggle, and so on. Hypnosis will help you improve the way you relate about yourself, not just by removing derogatory self-talk but also by promoting constructive self-reinforcing self-talk. It will have a knock-on impact on anything from self-confidence to decision-taking to job achievement.

Our implicit feelings may be passionate advocates, encouraging us to feel confident about the way we appear and our skill. Or the unconscious may be a harsh opponent who fills our heads with pessimistic, toxic feelings regarding us. The truth is: It is a serious struggle to conquer such pessimistic feelings.

Such feelings are profoundly rooted and ingrained in our brains. You peer through the reflection – and you bam! – The implicit one suggests you just don't like what you can see. It occurs naturally, unintentionally.

In other terms, poor self-esteem is sometimes the product of our latent deficiencies. Our unconscious mind is not logical. In reality, they are not focused – more much being rooted in adolescence – and they are also overly harsh and harmful.

And what if those feelings can be calmed or further yet, totally removed? Perhaps if we could just regain influence and teach our internal voice to be more compassionate, optimistic, and helpful? This is the foundation of the hypnotherapy for confidence. Through hypnosis, we reach these involuntary, subconscious thinking and try to unseat and re-frame them by the influence of imagination.

In brief, hypnosis may be an effective technique to target the root cause of poor self-esteem. It will help discourage certain cynical, unnecessarily positive feelings from asking us what to feel within us and motivating us to get rid of such pessimistic ways of thinking.

Our inner minds monitor our individual self-perceptions. And when harmful emotions are created, they can have an actual impact on our faith. Hypnotherapy tries to re-define these pessimistic self-conceptions and refresh some of them with good results. Hypnosis deals with identity-criticism, low self-confidence, poor self-esteem, self-consciousness, body dysmorphia, cynicism, uncertainty, and insecurity;

Smoking

It is not simple to give up the smoke. There are other ways to support you in quitting, such as prescribed drugs or nicotine gum. Studies show that people have discovered that therapy has enabled them to break the problem of smoking. Smoking reduction hypnosis operates well if you are practicing directly with a therapist who will refine the hypnosis treatments to fit your personality.

How it works is very interesting. You ought to genuinely decide to stop smoking in addition to hypnotherapy to succeed for quitting smoking. Hypnosis may be successful in two forms. One is to help you identify a safe, successful alternative practice, and then to direct your mind into the habit instead of smoking. This might be like eating a gum slice or heading for a stroll. The second is to prepare the subconscious to equate cigarettes with unpleasant stimuli, such as a poor flavor in the mouth or a disgusting scent of smoke.

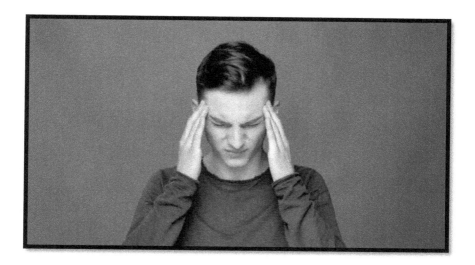

Chapter 2: Self-Hypnosis – The Ultimate Cure For Overthinking

Do you get caught in the head, contemplating your own emotions, suggestions, and events? Do you waste a lot of time worrying while you are going through life? This overthinking is very common for many of the world's population. Our capacity to actively perceive is one of the greatest attributes, as living beings. Our frontal lobes are so elaborately formed that stuff like planning and evaluation is a part of the routine, and we can carefully reflect on the world. Instead of doing the stuff you are supposed to do, when you worry so hard, you are said to be overthinking. Rather than behaving, you overthink as you evaluate, complain, and echo the very same thinking over and over again.

That habit stops you from acting. It uses up the energy, disengages your decision-making ability, and keeps putting you on a cycle of thought processes and thinking. This is a kind of mindset that is draining your time and resources and stopping you from doing, learning new stuff, and creating changes with your life. It is like binding oneself to a cord that is attached to a pillar and walking back and forth in loops. There's more possibility of stress, fear, and loss of inner harmony in this case. On the other side, when you overanalyze, you'll become more productive, more comfortable, and happier.

In this chapter, we will talk about the basics of overthinking, its telltale signs, and what is the psychology behind it. We will also look at the three types of overthinking along with its detrimental effects on our mental and physical health. Lastly, the chapter will end with a self-hypnosis script that you can follow at home before sleeping, some mindfulness tips, and a list of helpful daily affirmations to find calm.

2.1 Overthinking – A Modern Curse?

People sometimes go to doctors saying something like, "I can't sleep. It's like my brain won't turn off" or "I can't stop worrying that my life would have been much easier if I had handled something differently." A chicken-or-egg style problem is a connection between overanalyzing and mental health issues. Mental illnesses, such as anxiety and depression, are related to overthinking.

It's possible that overthinking leads emotional well-being to degrade, and the most inclined you become to overthink, the more your psychological health decreases. This is a deadly fall downwards. But, when you are stuck in the center of it, it's difficult to recognize the loop. Your brain can actively seek to persuade you that stressing and dwelling are beneficial in any way.

After all, if you invest enough time studying, would you not find a new approach, or keep yourself from falling into the exact same trap? In addition, most often, the reverse is valid. Paralysis in analyzes is a serious concern. The longer you talk about it, the worse you look. And your emotions of pain, fear, or frustration can affect your judgments and keep you from doing something constructive.

Overthinking appears in two ways; fixating about the mistakes and dreaming about the future. It is distinct from problem-solving. Problem-solving requires dreaming of a solution. To overthink implies focusing on the problem. Overthinking is distinct from self-reflection too. Good self-reflection means thinking about oneself or having a different outlook on a circumstance. It is purposive. Overthinking is about focusing on how awful you look and thinking of all the stuff you don't have influence. It isn't going to help you gain fresh knowledge. The distinction between problem-solving, self-reflection, and overthinking is not just how much energy you're spent in reflective thinking. It is beneficial to spend time finding new ideas to benefit your actions. But overthinking time, whether it's ten minutes or hours, isn't going to improve your life.

Signs of Overthinking

If you are more conscious of the propensity to overthink stuff, you may take measures to improve them. But first, you will realize that overanalyzing causes more damage than healthy. Often people believe that perhaps their overthinking impedes negative stuff happening. And they believe they would face more issues if they don't care sufficiently or rehash the experience sufficiently soon, anyway. Yet the work is fairly clear —- overanalyzing is terrible for you, and does little to avoid or fix issues.

The following are the signs that you are an overthinker.

1. You face difficulty pursuing and responding to dialogue as you go through possible answers or comments time and time again before the discussion has already concluded or the chance of an opportunity to talk has been closed-constantly contrasting yourself to the others around you and how you match up to them-Focusing on worst-case situations that include only your own

2. Overthinkers all too well realize how painful it is to fall asleep. Insomnia takes hold of you because you do not appear to be able to turn off your subconscious, so you are gradually overwhelmed with thinking. The mind runs, and you sound too activated to sleep; all of the day's concerns leave the mind flowing so you cannot avoid this emotional cage.

3. Another sign is living in terror. When you are living in fear of the unknown, then you are probably stuck in your head. Researchers noticed in a study that this anxiety is forcing the overthinkers to resort to opioids or drink to suppress their suicidal thoughts.

4. You overanalyze everything. One big issue with overthinkers is that they have a desire to monitor everything. They try to prepare for the future, but that is giving them tremendous fear because they cannot foresee it. Moreover, they don't want to do something they can't manage. We are deeply fearful of the unpredictable, which leads them to stay and think through all possibilities rather than act.

5. You get frequent headaches. You definitely worry too hard, whether you suffer from frequent headaches. Migraines signify that we should have a break of our bodies, and that requires relief from our own brains. Often, because you pay

careful attention to the feelings, you typically worry again and again on the same stuff.

6. You have an inability to live in the current moment. If you are not only willing to remain in this moment and appreciate life as it unfolds, then you're a target of overthinking. Too much thought allows you to lose perspective on the world around you, and get lost in your head. Becoming embroidered with thoughts separates you from the moment, which can interrupt your interaction with others.

7. When you choose to disregard the feelings of your heart and make lengthy lists of pros and cons. You will overthink it. Don't look at the advantages and disadvantages but let the heart chime in.

8. You are always fatigued. It also calls for a plan of action on our side as we are constantly exhausted. The bodies allow us to turn in to respond to their messages, rather than running from one thing to the next continuously to avoiding their requests. While tiredness may also be induced through doing too much and not sleeping, overthinking may also contribute to exhaustion. Consider this now (but not very much, of course): you don't allow your mind a break because you're always worrying about stuff. You can't work your mind 24/7; ultimately, you can get burned out.

9. A strong indication that you are overanalyzing is that you spend plenty of time obsessing on stuff that occurred in the past (going back to the same old topic in your head). You pick up events and experiences in your memory that could have occurred last night or maybe many years ago, and yet you're already talking about it, "psychologists claim. It's stressful. You're losing your mental resources worrying about it, so that may leave you feeling emotionally and mentally exhausted.

2.2 Psychology Of Overthinking

Our ideas can be steered at any specified point in life in a way that our perspective of that same set of situations changes from vibrant and sunny into shadows and cloudy. Take the first date, for instance. A minute later, "I'm so thrilled about this guy," we might say, "I wonder why he didn't call me yet," the thinking transforms. "Wasn't he really getting into me?"

And so, when we're sliding down the downward slope of overplaying, our heads are packed with assaults like" He was just a douche anyway. Nobody's going to be involved in me somehow. So why give it a try? "This is a clear illustration since most of us can feel connected to the chaotic tangle of emotions that enter our heads in the initial stages of a friendship, view, and over-analyze matching tone communications, and decipher ambiguous emojis. And the issue of overthinking spreads into other aspects of our lives. Even though spending time in deliberation is a crucial component of being a thoughtful, curious and self-conscious person capable of growth and change, lost time in pessimistic rumination nevertheless reinforces a cycle of self-limiting, self-destructive thinking and behavior.

People often get into problems when they get anxious. A UK Research of over 30,000 individuals have shown that fixating on traumatic events (particularly by personal-blame and overplaying) can be the best indication of some of today's most prevalent mental health problems. Most of the time, we overthink we focus on a negative thought process that leads to adverse outcomes. We listen in our minds to what Dr. Lisa Firestone, co-author of "Conquer the Vital Inner Dialogue," refers to as an "inner critical voice," relating to the detrimental facets of a scenario. This "speech" is like a psychopathic coach feeding us an endless flux of feedback and weakening our goals. That sensation arises as we are about to head to a work interview: "You'll never get this. You will get in shame andembarrassment. Just see how depressed you are. "As you focus on your partnership in your mind, it's the dialogue that is currently playing:" Why is she so cold and distant today? I must have already done something stupid. She is losing interest in me. She needs that one.'

Fear is the reason we overthink everything. During our youth, anxiety is triggered by thinking. We were not created with dread; however, it occurs either by social programming, life events, or trauma. Unluckily, we have very little or no control over what was learned to attribute to us in the times of our infancy. Most of us already have divisions of fear that have existed inside us since our days of childhood. Stuff happens to us in our youth, in our communities, our partnerships, and jobs, and the dark side of experiences is affecting us too hard. Feelings regarding these past interactions arise in a single minute of "thinking so much" like cumulative toxins seeping into the brain. We develop the harmful cycles of thinking that become almost unavoidable until we begin. We consider and ponder something that may be a perfectly harmless possibility, but this horror is produced as the toxin has burst and infiltrated our minds. The more we overcomplicate, the more and more fear we let in, and the more upsetting our thoughts are, particularly for those suffering from a fear condition, depression, and even thoughts of suicide. It's an indecisive loop.

In Decision Making Process Paralysis, the issue of Analysis Paralysis is an extremist-pattern or a condition of over-thinking or over-thought of a circumstance such that an intervention or judgment is never made, paralyzing the result. Ann individual with thinking paralysis gets so stuck in the cycle of analyzing and examining numerous data needed to make a judgment that they cannot act. Paralysis of analyzes occurs because we overanalyze when we have to make a decision.

It is essential to consider how our choice-making mechanism functions in order to fully understand the source of stagnation of the study. As per psychologist named Herbert Simon, we make choices and take action in one of two ways:

• Plenty of us, when making decisions, "Satisfy." It implies people who fulfill prefer the first option that fulfills their needs (or opt for an option that appears to fulfill more of their needs).

• Though some of the "maximize" the decision making process. Such citizens never compromise for the current option but keep on searching for new, stronger solutions.

For the two groups, maximizers are those that are prone to postpone judgment-making in the expectation for discovering,

offering, or selling a viable option, and who also suffer from thinking paralysis. Those are the men who overanalyze about success to come along.

In reality, some of us are using overthinking as default security. When we are forced to behave or make a judgment in fear of making a bad option, we over-analyze as a means to delay or stop our decisions. Psychologist Barry Schwartz originated the term "Paradox of Choice" to describe his simple observations that while expanded competition makes us achieve better outcomes statistically, it often contributes to greater fear, indecision, confusion, and deceit.

In today's modern era, if we have to make a decision, we are faced with an enormous and anxiety-inducing volume of data. Regardless of inspiring us to make smart decisions, our nearly limitless exposure to knowledge often contributes to a greater apprehension of doing the wrong option and taking the wrong judgment, which in effect causes us to run our heads in an almost unimaginable limbo of repetition of thinking or lack in consideration while going nowhere with essential tasks.

We are overthinking, and we are poor people seeking answers. We want certitude, and we like to be in charge. Don't stress! It is a practical aspect of human life. Okay, a little.

Probability theory involves an analysis of the potential consequences of an occurrence to decide what might actually happen in any particular circumstance.

Overanalyzing relates clearly to terror. Fear is the root of an ungodly flower. We have not been born with terror, but by imparted teachings, experience in life, or trauma, this fell upon us. Sadly, in the times of our youth, we have little to no influence on what was learned to given to us. Most of us already have divisions of terror that have been residing inside us since our childhood days. Stuff happens to us in adolescence, families, friendships, and work, and the negative aspect of interactions grip too firmly to us, feelings regarding these past encounters emerge like accumulated poison oozing into the mind in a single second of "doing so hard."

We shape certain damaging patterns of thinking, which are almost inevitable once we continue. We dream and talk of doing something that may be a perfectly harmless scenario, but that is because the toxin has exploded and invaded our brains that we are producing this world. The more we overthink, the more anxiety we allow in, and the more our emotions are disturbing. Particularly for those struggling from anxiety, illness, anxiety, and even suicidal thinking, it is a constant spiral. We know what it is like; before a major event, we worry too hard about it, we build imaginary beginnings and ends and even climaxes to the occurrence before it ever happens. It's planning, in a sense, so that we can live with whatever consequence there is and not struggle so badly from an unexpected event. We can't forecast the future, but inside us, there is a profound hope that we would have wishes.

Our experience helps one to do it half-way. In this way, we will sense that something is wrong, where we should or shouldn't go who we should and cannot trust. We have a strong voice within us which can save our lives at times. Overthinking blasts the sound. It's a difficult phase to go through, but sometimes it's required.

Rather than motivating us to make smarter decisions, our nearly unrestricted exposure to knowledge also contributes to greater anxiety of taking the wrong decision, which in effect causes us to spin our wheels in an almost inescapable purgatory of intellectual stagnation, all the while going nowhere on our essential ventures.

Analysis paralysis or stagnation by thought is a non-pattern, the process of over-examination (or overthinking) of a condition such that a judgment or intervention is never made, in essence, paralyzing the outcome. Our minds have a particular way of interpreting the universe and adapting to it than logical thinking. If we don't use these other forms of thinking for any purpose and needed to depend solely on empirical analysis, we may run into the question of lower returns.

This implies that the more you plan, the less profit you receive, the more you move beyond a certain point. Though it always seems helpful, it is ineffective. An individual suffering paralysis of thought gets so stuck in the cycle of assessing and reviewing specific evidence required to make a judgment that they cannot function.

If you are always planning ahead, while rarely take any initiative, then you are likely to be caught in the inertia of thought. Paralysis in analyzes is the process of over-thinking over judgment to the extent that a choice is never made.

It's cool to absorb information because if you don't do something about it, it's useless. Whether you're always asking whether you understand enough or not, you'll long wait.

So why do we harbor this internal adversary who feeds back such negative remarks and terrible advice on us? Here's one of the two reasoning: We all have two types of selves. We're just split into our true selves and our anti-selves.

While our true self is life-affirming, goal-driven, and represents our real values and expectations, our anti-self is like an internal enemy who is self-denying and auto-critical, cynical, and suspicious to both us and others. Our real or actual self is established from positive experiences in life, safe formative events, and the traits we encountered via our family members and early care providers. The anti-self is conditioned by the traumatic interactions, harmful incidents, and actions we've been exposed to early in life. For example, if we had a mother that did not consider us as nice, our pessimistic inner monologue would possibly mimic this unkind disposition toward us. We proceed to self-parent as adults, instructing the same stuff we were instructed as infants. If we stand shoulder to shoulder with our anti-self and pay attention to our voice of opposition within, this will lead us away to a traumatic path that is not based on reality. We may engage in a dangerous cycle of rumination, a type of negative thinking associated with depression, and perhaps even suicidal ideation.

Our parents have a contradictory feeling towards themselves as anyone else: they have strong feelings of optimistic self-consciousness, but often they even sound self-critical or identity-hating. Just as parents feel good and pessimistic about themselves, they often have sensitive, affectionate feelings and important responses to their babies. They have both the capacity to love and nourish their kids, yet they also have feelings of anger or rage. Since negative emotions for kids are both intimate and socially inappropriate, caregivers are not likely to consider and seek to ignore or hide such feelings within themselves. However, the detrimental aspect of the parents' ambivalence is expressed in both constructive acts and punitive attitudes that are particularly reactive to adolescents, and that leads to conflict inside the personalities. The child readily assimilates the positive attitudes of the parents and becomes part of the real self, while the child internalizes the negative attitudes of the parents as a foreign dimension into the personality, and becomes part of the anti-self.

The self-system, or real self, is composed of the unique characteristics of the individual, including biological, temperamental, and genetic characteristics, and its harmonious assimilation of the parents' positive attitudes and traits. This begins to grow as a consequence of the parents' affection and nursing, and also their way to fix the inevitable disturbances in parent-child intimacy. The outcomes of continued personal growth, schooling, and amplification of

good role models throughout a person's life make a contribution to the evolution of the self-system.

The ego-system comprises of the individual's desires — the essential requirements for nutrition, water, safety, and sex; the need for social contact, satisfaction, and lives-affirming behavior; the manifestation of affection, compassion, sympathy, and divine ambitions to find purpose in life — all are aspects of the ego-system. Positive long term factors allow the emerging person to develop and implement their own system of values and reinforce their capacity to live a decent life, that is to say, in accordance with their moral principles.

The anti-self mechanism is the personality's defense aspect; it derives from two sources, (1) from the internalization of parental aggression, and (2) as a preventive reaction to the negative side of parents' ambivalence: their rejection, hostility, indifference, and irresponsibility. Additionally, psychological starvation, over-protective attitudes, and lack of comprehension of a child's nature have a detrimental effect on its growth. Some mother and father unknowingly dispose of the attributes they dislike in themselves by reflecting them into their kids, and their kids integrate these definitions as a part of a detrimental self-concept or anti-self system.

The anti-self process arises as a consequence of the child's innate insecurity, hereditary propensity, gene expression conditions, temperament, and aversive influence on the world that might occur earlier in life (birth injury, disabilities, illnesses, painful breakups, and the possible loss of a family member or friend). The anti-self process is made up of defensive lines created in the family due to attachment issues and emotional trauma, which are later strengthened and exacerbated by the cognitive awareness of death in the child. The anti-self process is also influenced throughout one's lifetime by the misery related to the human condition (e.g., starvation, financial crisis, brutality, environmental catastrophes, disease, mental and physical degradation, and death).

The anti-self structure consists of the base safety, the fairytale relationship, or the personality-parenting process that involves self-nurturing and self-punishment tendencies. Ego-nurturing, ego-relieving inclinations are expressed via allegedly welcoming ego-protective, and/or self-regarding ideas and unhealthy impulses. Self-punishment tendencies are manifested in the dissenting voices inside and self-defeating, self-destructive behavioral patterns. The defense level is equal to the level of harm incurred when growing up as a kid up.

The two structures, self, and anti-self shape completely independently, and both are complex, constantly developing, and changing over time.

Many Americans are acquainted with the word mental illness (and, in reality, everyday millions and millions of people are suffering from any type of anxiety condition), but we appear to ignore a significant mental disorder symptom that is overthinking.

The concept of overplaying is something to ruminate or worry about. A lot of people may assume they are overthinkers after hearing this description. Who just doesn't go a mere day without trying to overthink something? We worry if we are making the correct decisions from little items like choosing the shortest path every morning on our drive or finding the best place for lunch to items like the well-being of our children and the health and well-being of our families. But it is natural. To some degree, it is normal to fear and to overthink.

There are, however, adverse consequences that overthink may have on an individual psychologically and physically. That will be repetitive thoughts on something that triggers one discomfort, pain, terror, or despair while overthinking when it relates to an anxiety disorder. It's not only so much thought about it-it's so obsessed about it that it damages one's ability to work throughout their life.

If you're concerned or stressing regarding yourself, your job, your kids, your mates, or something else, so you may not have an anxiety problem, what you've been thinking about, you're stressed for a moment, and you're moving ahead about your day in a brief amount of time. Often you tend to think, so you don't ruminate endlessly. You notice the stress doesn't mess with the entire life. However, with overplaying as a consequence of an anxiety condition, the concern becomes everything that the individual may care about, and while they do not struggle about the same problem all of the time, they are still worried about everything.

One explanation we overanalyze is that they make choices. Often, it's a huge call. Some moments, rather dumb decision-making, is about something, like what cafe to choose. Although you need to think of your choices, it's time to overthrow them, particularly if you have plenty of people queuing on you to make a decision.

2.3. Impact Of Overthinking On Health

Overthinking affects your emotional and physical health.

Overthinkers are more vulnerable to fear, depression, and other mental well-being problems. That is attributed to the fact that the emphasis on bad thoughts and reactions is continuous, which allows them to hang on even though nothing is wrong. To hold your emotional well-being in order, consider keeping the mind on positive feelings. It does influence the balance of the hormones.

Concentrating your attention on unpleasant emotions will disrupt the hormone equilibrium in your body and wear down the neurotransmitters required to feel good. Persisting on emotions of despair and frustration allows these molecules to deplete more quickly, which may cause depression. It may also induce hypertension and heart disease.

Thinking continually about the pressures of your life will trigger your blood pressure to increase. High blood pressure may contribute to a number of health issues, such as harm to the lungs and hypertension, which can even cause a stroke. It may be triggering intestinal disorders.

Overthinking will also impact the digestive tract. You will lead yourself to have irritable bowel syndrome (IBS) by overwhelming yourself with worrying about your issues constantly. IBS signs cause discomfort in the belly, cramping, nausea, and indigestion. Stressing oneself by overthinking will even contribute to ulcers in your stomach. These negative effects of overthinking will be discussed later down below.

Lately, research has accepted the idea that not just your emotional well-being but often, your physical health increasing be influenced by your feelings and thoughts. Openly felt and expressed emotions and opinions tend to float fluidly with no judgments or relation, without affecting our health. On the other side, repressed (particularly nervous or negative) feelings and overthinking will drain our mind of its strength, adversely impact the body and lead to physical health issues. It is important to recognize our patterns of thinking and emotions, and also to be aware of the implications they have — not only on one another but also on our parts of the body, behaviors, and relationships.

Negative feelings and feelings of worthlessness and frustration may produce constant stress that disturbs the body's hormone cycle, destroys the brain chemicals that are required for pleasure, and destroys the immune response. Chronic tension is literally raising our lifespan. Research has now demonstrated that tension shortens our DNA strands' 'end caps,' known as telomeres, which lead them to age more rapidly. Poorly controlled or repressed anger (hostility) is often related to a plethora of health problems such as elevated blood pressure (hypertension), stomach diseases, respiratory disease, and infection.

Although it is really tempting to struggle over things beyond your grasp, to overthink is never a healthy habit to fall into. In the previous parts of the chapter, it has been discussed that focusing on the negative will create problems in your career, personal and emotional life, but sadly the practice of overplaying just doesn't end there. It has some significant consequences for well-being too. Here are several aspects in which overthinking will screw with your well-being in health and well-being.

1. Mental health: Anxiety, depression, or other mental health problems are more susceptible to overthinkers. This is because the focus on bad thoughts and emotions is constant, causing them to ruminate. A 2013 research released in the Journals of Behavioral neuroscience reported that dwelling on your shortcomings, errors, and issues raises the chance of mental health disorders. Rumination will set you up for a revolving circle, which is hard to crack. Ruminating creates emotional health chaos. Your propensity to fixate is increasing, with your psychological health declining.

2. Hormone deficiency: Concentrating the mind continuously on unpleasant feelings will disrupt the body's hormone balance and disintegrate the chemicals in the brain required to feel good. The emotions of desperation, despair, and anger cause these hormones to deplete faster and may contribute to depression and other body-related hormone imbalances.

3. Hypertension and heart disease: Excessive thinking about your life's issues can trigger your blood pressure to increase. High blood pressure can lead to a range of health issues, such as arterial injury and hypertension, and may also cause a stroke. Chest discomfort, lightheadedness, and tachycardia are some of the common risks you can encounter when you overthink obsessively.

4. Digestive system illnesses: The digestive tract may also be impaired by overthinking. You will cause irritable bowel syndrome (IBS) by constantly straining yourself with fretting about your issues. Symptoms of IBS include stomach discomfort, diarrhea, cramping, and cramping. Worrying yourself by overanalyze will even contribute to stomach ulcers. Certain gastrointestinal conditions such as IBD, i.e., inflammatory bowel disease, alterations in gastrointestinal motility and gastrointestinal mucus, decreased intestinal

permeability, and improvements in the intestinal micro-biota can often result in stress sensitivity.

5. Poor immune response: Overthinking can wear your immune function down, and can hamper your ability to combat even the flu virus. In the end, a poor immune system will lead you to have certain severe illnesses.

6. Cognitive Functions: Work suggests people believe they are healing themselves by rehashing their concerns through their heads. Results, therefore, demonstrate that the disability state of the experiment is true. The over-analysis of all in existence severely plays havoc with issue-solving skills. Rather than seeking answers, it will allow you to dwell on the problem. When you're an over-thinker, even the easy choices, like selecting how to dress for an event, or determining where to go on holiday, may seem like a choice involving life or death. Alas, all that contemplation won't help you make a smarter choice.

7. Sleep Disturbance: If you're an over-thinker, you possibly already realize you can't comfortably rest and sleep at night because your mind won't be turning off. Studies affirm that finding fixating and agitation contributes to fewer hours of sleep. You'll be more apt to twist and switch for hours before

slipping on. But sleeping later cannot benefit because overanalyzing hinders the standard of sleep. Since thinking over the same issue over and over again, you would be less likely to slip into a deep sleep. When you can't relax, you'll be pacing your mind, and you might have anxious feelings of going to sleep. Often, such overanalyzing occurs while there is exhaustion, and the next day starts. You feel exhausted, and you feel less concentrated. You may have persistent and pessimistic feelings about not sleeping. To exactly this cause insomnia is called a period of viciousness. It's impossible to avoid overthinking while you're an insomniac overthinking over not sleeping.

8. Skin Issues: Excessive fear, stress, and overthinking impacts the face. Different skin conditions such as rosacea, urticaria, contact dermatitis, hair loss, seborrheic dermatitis can be exacerbated or even worsened by overthinking-induced emotional tension. Stress triggers systemic inflammation and triggers flare-ups of the skin. Chronic stress that is induced by rumination impacts the intricate integrated skin structure, the adrenal glands, and the immune response, which aggravates skin diseases.

9. Cancer risk: Overthinking leads to stress and excessive activation of the hypothalamic-pituitary-adrenal axis impairing immune responses, which lead to the development and progression of some cancers.

10. Brain Fatigue: This requires a lot of emotional resources to overthink. Your subconscious produces too many various ideas and circumstances that are not necessarily directed for positive stuff. Without some physical source, emotional strength can leave you completely wasted and making you look like you're tired because you've spent too long in your own mind. Our brains, as we overthink, contain cortisol, the stress hormone, we stress ourselves out. Over time, the continuous release of cortisol will deplete and induce burnout. It is like pushing the car with the wrong gear. The engine is going so you're not getting too far.

11. Appetite changes: Overthinking may have a detrimental impact on people's appetites. For others, it can reduce appetite, and it can improve appetite for others — which is more popular. That's called "worried food," so people do it because it's soothing, or even calming. Most people prefer to reach for the tastiest yet most harmful things while they're afraid to overthink, so there's an explanation that high-fat, sugar items are called "comfort foods." However, according to

Harvard University, cortisol — the stress hormone — increases the appetite together with the desire to consume junk food.

To consider workable options helps to learn about an issue. Yet those that fixate don't get this done. Without providing remedies, they continually talk about the reasons for and effects of their issues. We might not really realize we are just fixating. They may believe they're trying to understand, obtain knowledge, solve issues, and decode events' broader significance. Truth is nothing to overthink gets resolved. If your emotions incapacitate you, growing more anxious and exhausted by the passing of time, then realize that you may unknowingly ruminate or overthink in an unreasonable way.

2.4 Sleep Hypnosis – The Magic Wand For Overthinking And Anxiety

While hypnotherapy is not so well recognized as psychotherapy and anxiety management medicine, for many years, scholars and scientists have been researching the impact it may have on mental health problems such as anxiety, overthinking, post-traumatic stress disorder (PTSD), and insomnia. Researchers examined people's brains in one 2016 research as they were attending controlled sessions of hypnosis. They find that a hypnotized brain encounters brain changes that offer an individual the following:

- Less insecurity

- Paying closer attention

- Greater regulation over the physical and mental aspects

Let's just assume you are scared to ride. The psychiatrist will send you what's recognized as a "posthypnotic idea" during a therapy session when you're in a trance state. The mental is more accessible to suggestion in this fantastical condition. This helps the psychiatrist to say how quickly you'll feel comfortable when you get on a plane each time.

If you're in a calm environment, it may be harder to resist worsening the signs of distress that you can have, such as:

- Breathlessness

- Muscular pain

- Increasing heart rhythm

- A sense of imminent despair

- Nervous tummy

- Irritability

Hypnotherapy is thought to be an alternative to cognitive-behavioral treatment. If you use hypnotherapy to relieve the fear, it may have comparable results to that in meditation. An entrancing relaxation, much like mindfulness, will help place you in this calm condition. This condition will instead be used to treat anxieties and mental illnesses.

And, if you're attempting to overcome anxiety about the flight, you might see yourself heading straight to the first moment you've been terrified to travel. You may use a strategy called Hypno-projectives, where you visualize what you would have loved to see in the previous activities. And in the future you will see yourself, feeling relaxed and peaceful whilst on a boat.

What do we do when we realize we can actually profit from maintaining a state of consciousness, but we feel unable to do so; when we lose the drive to do it as we have missed the strength to take the next move forward? For these cases, the application of sleep hypnotherapy always works. Of starters, maybe there's a thought leader that encourages you to listen to them on video or audio, a chapter of a novel you've never read that has had an impression on your experience, or a song you might respond to.

It is a means of going into a state of consciousness guided by someone else and their teachings. This behavior needs minimal mental energy and no other physical activity than pressing on a button. So listening to any audio-awareness in a case like this is very effortless and normal.

Audio hypnosis is good for this. Yes, mindfulness and hypnotherapy are related and share certain parallels, as a condition of consciousness is close to the state of mind that you are in while you are guided by a sound in a hypnosis session. Sleep hypnosis will reach out to us on an unconscious basis. The subconscious controls our lives. It is a reflection of all that we have learned in practice, which is accountable for our views, which assessment on ourselves and the environment around us.

And if we alter our underlying values, our behaviors would shift and how we cope with challenges in life. This ensures that entering a state of consciousness and having a more "awakened" and conscious attitude to the challenges of life is even simpler for us. Emotional challenges function far better on the "feeling stage" than the "thought stage," which is why it is so important to learn and think positively while struggling to deal with anxiety, insecurity, low self-worth feelings, and pessimistic thoughts. You may use hypnosis to help you feel better, which also helps you think of a problem differently. For the future, though, hypnosis promotes positive behavioral actions.

Although self-hypnosis, which is the form of listening to audios through hypnosis, is typically aim-oriented and used to resolve anxiety, cure depression, and assist through problems with self-confidence, etc., it is definitely also well adapted to the practice with mindfulness. Indeed, if we look at meditation rituals across the centuries, we do see a variety of hypnotic activities like singing, mantra recitals, praying, vocals, and listening to hypnotic sounds like Tibetan bowls and chimes. Please note that in the conventional context, you don't need to meditate to participate in meditation on mindfulness. There are numerous avenues to regain, so to say, the mind to move it to the core back into a condition of present consciousness.

Throughout the practice of mindfulness, we devote our complete focus to one topic at a time as a means to teach our brains to be open to another level of perception, "under" the discursive brain & cognitive consciousness (what the hypnotist calls executive operations) and indeed, the calming mechanism of the amygdala may be triggered and conditioned, for example, via active, focused breathing. In this sense, meditation reflects the receptiveness of hypnosis.

In hypnotherapy, one is guided and shown how to slip below the wave of conditioned cycles of thought and interpretation to a responsive, accessible condition in which ideas from the practitioner may be integrated and transformed into conscious experience. We're doing something close but still something special. We may often evoke the calm, aware, responsive altered condition, but we prioritize analysis, questioning, and an in-depth look at what occurs (intending to consider rather than condemn, and welcoming, non-judgmental method in hypnosis is similar).

Humans make efforts to create meaning of our issues with our usually busy, multi-tasking brains to continue and watch a film when at the same moment, another wants to carry on a discussion with you. Both the film and the dialogue that make some sense on their own terms, but combined, they are a mess of contradictory and confounding elements that feel utterly daunting and, at times, threatening. The practice of carefulness (and therapy) helps the person to acquire the attitudinal skills to experience this confusion and react calmly and politely, and the sensitive skills to guide focus (and relational resources) to the "actual" problems and likely away from those perceived or expected. This change will encourage a person to see things for what they really are and to understand that the concepts and tales we all make are just this: inventions and not truths that need to be discussed or resolved.

Explain hypnosis allows your direct exposure to your mind's imagination – the unconscious, which is the key. It is here where your "real name" rests. Everything that represents who you truly are, always remain inside the unconscious. And the reason hypnotherapy makes you return to your internal "playground" is the reason it stimulates the thinking mind.

To put it better, assume there was a gatekeeper who stopped you from peering through the archives and libraries of the subconscious mind to make sure you didn't get too far in the way. So this gatekeeper is involved in via hypnosis. And if the gatekeeper is distracted, a hypnotherapist will also explore the unconscious foundations.

Thus hypnosis and trance only unlock the screen. They encourage you to completely envision how far better life will be (often in vibrant Technicolor detail), what it will feel

possible to adopt entirely different attitudes, values, and personalities.

Despite this, the one aspect that hypnosis provides is that other common day treatments are missing is the opportunity to silence their own stressful communications. Have you ever thought that you'd try to see a meaningful improvement, only to have a reasonable mind of yours wake up to remind you that you can't? It's the secret emotional conversation that most treatments don't appear to be creeping through. Hypnosis is doing a great job of deflecting this. Another aspect that distinguishes hypnosis is the capacity to reorganize mental illusions.

Hypnosis causes thought, passive, and involuntary cognitive illusions and destructive ego-schema to be viewed and restructured (altering the template). In case you question what the last word applies to – self-schema – it's the long-lasting and consistent collection of memories that makes up the convictions, perceptions, and assumptions regarding yourself in different behavioral realms. And it so occurs that, inevitably, hypnosis changes the ego-schema.

Those suffering from overthinking and fear are also afflicted with very pessimistic feelings. When you've been in the midst of a "run," how serious it will get is always hard to find out.

The morbid and skewed perception that follows anxiety and panic disorders will rob certain people of what will actually be an enjoyable day.

Re-framing helps an individual to get a different viewpoint (aka, in specific, placing a new screen around something). So let's look at what a structure is. A construct is a sense in which there is a concept or theory. The re-framing takes a turn backward and gives a new view. This is simply bringing the concept or theory into another form. To find more inventive solutions, it is a way of observing and understanding things, thoughts, beliefs, and feelings. Re-framing offers us the chance to find the ray of hope of otherwise hopeless circumstances. The significance that you add to a case relies on the beliefs you make regarding it (those are creeds, principles, etc.). All re-framing does is give up fresh life opportunities for the public to see and feel.

A Deep Sleep Hypnosis Script

1. Sit in a comfortable spot, peacefully. Know you may use self-hypnosis anytime, but diversion-free environments definitely improve concentration, particularly if you're new to the process.

2. Breathe in deeply, melodically, and gently for a few times. To the count of five, you might want to breathe in and breathe out deeply. Or inhale, hold for an instant, and start releasing for a lengthier exhale. Find something that feels most soothing to you. Close your eyelids if you have not done so already.

3. Imagine yourself in a position that will offer harmony and warmth. It doesn't have to be everywhere you ever were or even a particular place. On Jupiter, you might be riding a unicorn, if it soothes you. Or you could prefer a more everyday spot, like your bath or the beach. You could even make a happy recollection come back. Just isolate an enjoyable setting you'd like to spend a bit of time in.

4. Immerse all the sensations to keep you rooted in your current mental environment. Smell the apple pie household-recipe of your grandma, whether you've wanted to return the memories of your youth. Feel the wind of the ocean on your face and the sand between your feet as you visualize the beach. See the candlelight flicker in a soothing warm bath from your point of view.

5. Select affirmation that you know is required right now. Assurance can be customized to any situation is actually particulars or as basic as a few terms like, "I'm healthy" or "I'm

powerful." For flying anxiety, find a mantra that tells me that air transport is short, like "I'm going to be home early."

6. Play your affirmation echoed in your head, enabling them to fall deeper into it. Concentrate your efforts on making them believable. Live in this hypnotic condition as much as you want or as much as time is allowed.

2.5 Mindfulness Tips For Overthinking

Whenever you find yourself spiraling out of control with overthinking and rumination, follow these amazing mindfulness tips to be calmer, centered, and at ease.

1. Do a meditation practice or practice mindfulness

Meditation may be as easy as locating a sliver of room and launching an email. Apps and online programs are a great way to immerse your toe in practice without engaging in an expensive class or taking up a lot of time. Innumerable private, guided meditations are accessible online. Such Applications for Meditation are a perfect starting point.

2. Set an Intention

There's a purpose why the yoga instructor wants you to create a goal on the day for your workout. If you're reading so in the daily magazine right before big events, creating a goal will help you concentrate and remember why you're doing it. Set an intention for it if something gives you anxiety — like giving the big speech at work. You can set an intention anywhere to take care of your needs, for example, before heading to the gym or treat your body with compassion before feeding.

3. Focus on One Task at a Time

Sure, if you do it correctly, the to-do list may be a form of meditation. Set a five-minute timer, and send your complete and full attention to one mission. No scanning of the computer, no tapping on updates no web surfing-no multi-tasking at all. Let the one job come to the surface before the timer is off.

4. Turn Chores into a Mental Break

Instead of being distracted with your to-do list or clutter, just let yourself rest at the moment. Dance when you're preparing the plates, or reflect on how the cleaner flows through the walls when washing the tub. Take five deep breaths while waiting for the microwave to end. Fantasize while sorting the sheets.

5. Wish Bliss to Other Individuals

You only need 10 seconds from writer and former Google innovator Chade-Meng Tan to do that practice. I wish others to be content at random during the day. All of this exercise is in your mind. You only have to set the good energy. Check it out on the drive, at the workplace, at the fitness center, or while standing in line. Brownie points if you find yourself upset or annoyed with somebody, and you hold back and wish them happiness (mentally) instead. With eight nominations for the Nobel Prize, Meng may be onto anything.

6. Consider What May Go Well, Not What Can Go South

Overthinking is in several situations triggered by one particular emotion: panic. It's easy to get paralyzed when you concentrate on all of the adverse things that would happen. Next time you feel like you are spiraling in that course, pause. Visualize all the stuff that might go better and hold certain feelings upfront and current.

7. Journaling

Journal, no way is right and wrong. From using the organized 5-Minute Journal to jotting your mind on a random paper scrap, the act of writing it down can help relieve the mind and

cool spinning ideas. Attempt a list of thanks or actually pinpoint the three great things that have occurred today.

8. Appreciate Everything

You cannot all at the same time hold a remorseful thought and a happy thought, so why not use the moment in a constructive way? Create a note of what you are thankful for every morning, every evening. Have a friend with thanks and swap lists, and you'll have a testament to the positive stuff surrounding you.

One aspect that can happen to someone is overthinking. So if you have a perfect program to work with it, at least you can fend off any of the gloomy, nervous, overwhelming thoughts and transform this into something positive, constructive, and efficient.

9. Avoid Flawlessness

This one is tall. We should finally quit searching for those of us who are looking for greatness right now. Being positive is awesome, but it's impossible, unsustainable and crippling to reach for excellence. The minute you start thinking, "This must be flawless" is the minute you have to remember, "Waiting for the perfect is never as intelligent as making progress."

2.6 Mindfulness Affirmations

If your emotions are running and you do not appear to be able to get them under control, you can only help to say one or two affirmations to yourself. You will subdue the storm that is the head by repeating a short sentence again and again, and regain peace and order. You disrupt the looping transmission of electrons' thought patterns in your brain and force it back into a more balanced environment by replacing your hapless thoughts with a simple yet powerful affirmation.

- **Affirmations for Worries**

I look forward to having wonderful experiences in the future

I have the power of my own future.

For me, it's all happening in life.

I draw positive stuff into my life.

I'll accept all that happens, and accept it.

With bravery and wisdom, I'll confront any challenge.

I'll happily fix whatever tough problem.

I relinquish the need to control things.

All that happens to me is always good

I have the power to establish that life that I want.

- **Affirmations for Past Experiences**

I forgive all previous faults.

I accept all of that's transpired in my life so far.

The past has no influence or authority over me.

I thank myself for all my past experiences.

I am thankful for the learning experiences in my life.

I let go of issues and fears in the past.

I live in the current moment.

- **Affirmations to Calm Down**

I am safe from all the worries in the world.

I just let go of my anxiety and stress.

I'm cool, self-assured, and focused.

I really become a more confident person each day.

For me, it's easy to be relaxed.

I feel relaxed and calm.

My body feels comfortable.

- **Affirmations for Overthinking**

My mind is quiet, and I feel relaxed.

I live in the present moment.

I am overflowing with joy and peace.

I remove those bad feelings that aren't of use to me.

I hold my thoughts in order.

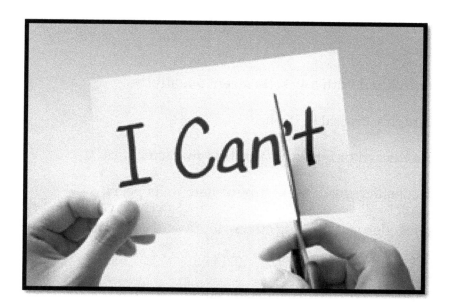

Chapter 3: Hypnosis To Boost Self-Esteem

Self-esteem is your own view. Individuals with good self-esteem respect their accomplishments. Although everybody sometimes loses trust, individuals with poor self-esteem may, most of the time, feel depressed or dissatisfied with them. This can be resolved, but to boost self-esteem requires care and daily practice.

An individual with low self-esteem usually:

- Is highly critical of itself

- Play down or ignore its positive characteristics

- It considers itself to be subordinate to its peers.

- Uses derogatory adjectives to describe them as dumb, obese, hideous or nasty

- Includes conversations with ourselves (this is called 'self-discussion') that are often pessimistic, unfair and accusing ourselves

- Presumes that fortune plays a big part in all their successes and does not take their credit

- Blames themselves when events go wrong instead of taking certain factors into consideration that they have little influence over, such as other people's behavior or economic powers

They don't trust anyone complimenting them.

This chapter will discuss the origins of how low esteem is developed in childhood and what are the other factors involved in it. Then, we will dig deeper into the power of our words and how negative self-talk damages our self-esteem and lowers confidence. Afterward, we will also dive into the ways we can develop positive self-talk. Lastly, the chapter will also highlight the benefits of sleep self-hypnosis to improve poor self-esteem along with a list of affirmations to cope with it.

3.1 How Is Low Self-Esteem Developed?

It is assumed that previous encounters shape both self-esteem and self-confidence. We get tons of unpleasant and optimistic feedback in life – which would have a big effect on how we think about ourselves. The reviews will originate from our friends, the media, and our families. And sadly, we become more sensitive and open to harmful signals-in the amygdala, they are far more likely to be tucked away. Trauma, too, will

adversely influence our self-esteem and self-confidence. Tragic events will undermine our self-esteem and our level of trust.

As a result, self-esteem is expressing itself on a graph. Some even have loads, whilst others can fail in some cases. Yet humans with poor self-esteem continue to have a persistent poor self-worth degree. They would most definitely witness and feel:

- Despair or sadness

- Boredom and lack of motivation

- Being unnecessarily responsive to critique

- Low assertiveness

- Hearing pessimistic, over-critical self-conversation

- Feeling that their lives had ended

We may establish adverse views about us, even quite early on in life: a traumatic social interaction, a mockery about our behavior, a loss of a study. Such interactions continue to impact our self-perception lastingly – well into our adult years.

Our unconscious, for example, needs to shield us. The amygdala creates defensive strategies after unpleasant interactions – i.e., starting to feel like you're terrible at holding discussions with new friends – to protect us from experiencing the pain, or guilt, or embarrassment that we may have felt. As such unconscious thinking, this security unfolds. Of starters, after that traumatic social interaction, your subconscious may have begun to warn you: You don't like social circumstances. You're not nice at them; you just should stop them. And the negative is becoming a prophecy which fulfills itself. They believe so compellingly that we would struggle to speak to potential friends that we would have a rough experience for ourselves, allow our shyness to hang on, and force ourselves to stop meeting other people.

If left unchecked, the low self-esteem and trust can cause us to continuously have such negative experiences. Therefore they are too difficult to eliminate. Since we have empowered the subconscious to decide how, over a period, we can feel towards ourselves and our talents, we encourage such feelings to be constantly enhanced.

Several of the reasons for low self-esteem could include:

- For example, inadequate treatment by a wife, adult or caregiver in an abusive situation

- Continued medical conditions such as persistent discomfort, severe disease or functional impairment

- Dissatisfied upbringing in which family (or other important individuals including educators) were highly negative

- Continued traumatic life events, such as a breakdown of relationships or financial hardship

- Low educational success at school contributing to a loss of trust

- A mental condition, such as anxiety or depressive condition.

Following are some of the other causes of low self-esteem in detail:

1. Unconcerned Caregivers

Motivating one to do better, aspiring for success, and believing that you merit more because your family or other key providers have not given notice – as though your biggest successes weren't deserving of mention. Perhaps this situation contributes to feeling overlooked, unrecognized, and subsequently irrelevant. It may even leave you thinking like you are not responsible to anybody, or you may assume that no one in the here and now is bothered about your location, but it's just thinking of past carry-over. Feeling unacknowledged will contribute to the conviction that you will apologize for your life.

2. Bullying (with Parents who are not supportive)

If you had a love of a fairly healthy, sensitive, conscious family, after being taunted and humiliated as a teenager, you would have had a stronger chance of healing and restoring your self-esteem. If you still feel insecure at home and torment persisted beyond your house, your daily existence became pervaded by the crushing feeling of being helpless, deserted, hopeless, and overflowing with self-loathing. It may also seem like someone who is friends with you does you a favor, when you see yourself as so hurt. Or you may believe that someone who is interested in your life needs to be dishonest and not trusted. Absent a healthy family environment, the consequences of abuse will be magnified, and the standard of living undermined miserably.

3. Traumatic Past

The most prominent and explicit triggers of poor self-esteem may be physical, psychological, or psychological violence. To be put against your desire into an emotional and physical situation will make it really difficult to appreciate the environment, trust oneself, or trust people, which have a significant impact on self-esteem. This could also seem like your responsibility though your guilt could not be any less. Obviously, there's so much going at one time in these scenarios that you may need to check out, disassociate, and go away. It can leave you feeling like nothingness. In an attempt to take ownership of the situation, you might have told yourself in the mind that you have been involved or perhaps to blame. You may have discovered strategies to deal with the violence, to handle the confusion in strategies you recognize to be toxic, and you can finally see yourself amid a zillion of other emotions as disgusting and seemingly disgraceful.

4. Belief Systems

If the spiritual (or other) set of values places you in a place of thinking as though you were constantly sinning, that may be comparable to dealing with a person of resentful authority. Whether judgments emanate from sources of power or from an existing set of values in your existence, it may elicit humiliation, remorse, tension, and self-loathing. There are two ways that many formal value structures offer: one that is all positive and one that is all evil. If you finally slip between the two into the pit, you end up feeling lost, misunderstood, disoriented, ashamed, false, and frustrated in one over and over.

5. Media and the Society

It's no secret that media people are packaged into unachievable scales of perfection and thinness and retouched into. It is an outbreak that just gets uglier. And both men and women fear like they cannot live up to what's out there. Perhaps the roots of poor self-esteem are sown everywhere, yet there is little escape from feelings of failure now that culture and the media find imperfections so readily available. When exposure to the media is accessible younger and younger, sooner and sooner, children are exposed to such false similarities.

Watching TV, searching online, or reading a paper may cause a flood of negative thinking, appearances, assets, or job. Having a fit, slim beauty getting berated for adding a few pounds would never make us feel happy! If you may and never ignore that the news and pictures that we use are always distorted, stop cynicism in the news.

6. Disapproving Adults

When you grew up thinking that everything that you did wasn't good quality, how can you mature into a person with a strong self-image? If you've been attacked no matter what you've achieved or how hard you've worked, it is hard to feel relaxed and secure later on in your own skin. The guilt that has been put upon you for constant "failure" will seem unbearable blindingly.

7. Bullying (with too supportive parents)

Alternatively, if your mother and father were overly supportive and unwarranted, it can make you feel poorly prepared for the harsh world. Without an initial reason for forming a thick outer coat, it may seem difficult and even embarrassing to see oneself as unwilling to deal with the pressures of life just outside of the house. From this point of view, you may feel unprepared and profoundly embarrassed to admit to your parents even this dirty hideous secret about you, because you have to defend them from the discomfort they would suffer if they realized. You concealed the horrible truth of what has occurred to you, instead. Shame will cloud the view. Ultimately it might feel as though the viewpoint of your family regarding you contrasts with the opinions of the community regarding you. It can force you to cling to what is familiar in your life, as it is difficult to trust what is real and what is not. You should doubt the legitimacy of the optimistic opinion that your parents have about you, and settle on the belief that you're not really good enough or victim-like, and will be the target about mockery.

The first principle of learning to accept and regard yourself is to remove poor self-talking from your repertoire altogether. Ego-criticism is very damaging, and you will never ever talk about yourself or to yourself in a disrespectful manner because all you do is train yourself about feeling worse. From time to time, we are all guilty of derogatory self-talk, and it's easy to get into the trap.

8. Being Humble

There is a propensity notably in Britain to 'dust off' praise. When anyone acknowledges your job, you may catch yourself transferring some else's credit. If anyone adores your dress, you might tell you've had one for years. Learn to acknowledge congratulations, wave, and tell thank you!

9. Early Conditioning

Because of previous learning, we sometimes tend to refer to ourselves in a derogatory way from others who have an effect over us, including families, educators, or even spouses. People who criticize others often find themselves trapped in their own issues of self-esteem, and need to bring others down in order to make them feel superior. Get over its bitterness.

3.2 Negative Self-Talk And Self-Esteem – The Power Of Words

Conventional hypnotherapy works by helping to ensure messages from the hypnotist are unquestionably accepted by the mental internal or unconscious part. To achieve so, the hypnotherapist will penetrate the rational mind-the gatekeeper. And she achieves so in a variety of forms-one of which is emphasizing the phrase frequently.

The recurrent messages that we obtain as kids help to form our self-esteem and self-confidence. Whenever people are in any kind of emotionally charged state, such messages have additional power if collected. And the frightened and sorrowful condition of that little kid rendered him particularly vulnerable to the reinforcement of the 'dumb, dumb' word. Such messages already have the powerful impact of hypnosis.

Fortunately, most of our unnecessary early life experiences or belief systems are weakened by experiences and circumstances and the passage of time, except if we unknowingly continue to hypnotize ourselves negatively. Do not pay attention to one's self-talk, the quiet chit chat that continues in one's head. Will this raise you up or destroy you?

You say 'you foolish, stupid 'boy/girl anytime you make an error. Will you silently side with them as somebody criticizes you as if it were just another evidence of your poor self-worth? Do you take on the pessimistic hypnotherapy of overstressed and frustrated teachers or of parents who are caring yet afraid and unqualified? Our comments on self-talking have a very strong impact on us. They are so repetitive, just like hypnosis, that we rarely question them.

They are persistent - and we are deliberately waiting to 'hear' them. And they're either so repetitive that we're lulled into embracing them actively, or really emotionally charged and affecting. Many individuals understand this and seek to stop this destructive self-hypnosis. Yet most of them go the opposite way through it-preferring not to speak about themselves. But let's be explicit about one issue-you're never going to stop talking yourself. Consider that, and you're halfway to stopping self-harm. What's more, a meaningful feature of your thought process is your self-talk. That needs addressing is what you say to your own selves.

One powerful but deceptively easy approach is to note the old messages and contest them. We raise their strength by giving legitimacy to them by pulling them through the light of day.

Back up that by dismissing their legitimacy: "Is this actually relevant now in my existence-all these decades later?"

In other terms, if you concentrate exclusively on the negative implications of a life incident, over extended stretches of time, you become more apt to revisit the unpleasant feelings and memories in your mind. This type of recurrent negative-thinking clouds the view and affects how you and you interact with the world. Low self-esteem is clearly a major result of poor self-talk, so people with low self-esteem prefer to outsource their bad emotions towards themselves, creating a number of other issues.

For starters, a 2005 research showed that low self-esteem leads to higher levels of violence — verbal as well as physical — against others. In Austin, the College of Texas Psychology and Behavioral Health Service states three key "types" of poor self-esteem, the forms in which individuals extend their pessimistic perceptions about oneself into the universe.

The first one is "The Imposter." The imposters appeared content and pleased with their lives on the surface, but they actually need achievement after the performance to preserve their self-satisfaction façade.

This might contribute to problems related to perfectionism, rivalry, and burnt-out feeling. Rebel forces reject executive power and accuse others of their behavior, but underneath it all, this is just because people felt they're haven't ever been good enough. They show this impression by declaring that the opinions of other people do not matter — all just too falsely claim that no one can harm them.

The last one is "The Victim." Victims sometimes wait on others to assist them in solving their issues as they feel that they are not able to deal with the world on their own, which may contribute to timidity, under-realization, and over-reliance in friendships with others. Sometimes they use self-blame or denial as reasons not to take care of their affairs.

Though all of these "names" uniquely suffer poor self-esteem, the consequences are about the same. Low self-esteem may trigger people to encounter difficulties with their friendships; adversely impact their success at work or in their classwork; raise their chances of depression; trigger high rates of tension, isolation, and insecurity and contribute to increased risks of substance and alcohol addiction. The worst thing is that both of these results strengthen the distorted perception still retained by individuals with poor self-esteem, locking them in a continuous loop of depression. Bad thought often induces emotions of powerlessness when dealing with difficult circumstances and may also inhibit the capacity to deal with tension in general, contributing to worse results that might cause more tension — yeah, you predicted it.

Negative thoughts have even proved to cause hypertension, even when you don't have negative thoughts at the moment. If you notice derogatory self-talking, there are a variety of ways you can improve your attitude. Firstly, finding places that require a shift in mentality is critical. Perhaps you are constantly worrying adversely about your work, or about your partnership or family.

Everyone has an inner critic. Often this little voice may really be supportive of holding us focused toward goals — like when this criticism tells us that what we're about to consume isn't safe, or what we're about to do-not be smart. However, sometimes this tiny voice may be dangerous rather than beneficial, especially when it comes to the domain of unnecessary criticism. It is called pessimistic self-talk, and it really does drag us down.

Negative self-talk is what most of us feel from moment to time, and in several cases, it arrives. It often causes tremendous discomfort, not only for us but for everyone around us, if we are not vigilant. Here's what you need to learn about harmful self-discussion and its impact on the body, mind, existence, and loved ones.

Negative self-expression can take different forms. It may sound anchored ("I'm not successful at this, so I will stop trying it out for my own self-defense," for instance), or it may sound simply symbolic ("I will never get it right!"). It can take on the appearance of being a rational evaluation of a scenario ("I've only got a" C "on this exam. I think I'm not good at physics."), only to transform into a guilt-based illusion ("I'll actually fail that class and will never go to a successful college."). The ramblings of your negative self-talk, or "internal judge," from your background may sound an awful lot like a critical parent or relative. It may pursue the course of traditional false beliefs: catastrophe, guilt, and the like. Negative self-talk is essentially any inner conversation you have with yourself that may hinder your desire to trust in yourself and your own talents and achieve your potential. You and your capacity to make changes that will help, or your self-belief in your capacity to do so is diminished by any thought. Because of this, not only can poor self-talk be frustrating, it can also really hinder your performance.

Poor self-talk may have some very detrimental impacts on us. A big-scale study showed that rumination and ego-blame about bad events were associated with an increased risk of mental health issues. Concentrating on bad feelings may result in lower morale as well as increased feelings of worthlessness. This kind of critical internal dialog has even been associated with depression, so it's certainly something to fix.

Many that often catch themselves involved in derogatory self-talking appear to get more depressed. That's mostly how their perception is modified to construct an environment where they may not have the opportunity to achieve the expectations they set for them. This is due both to a reduced capacity to see possibilities all over them, and a decreased propensity to rely on those opportunities. This suggests that the enhanced awareness of stress is also related to pure experience as well as the behavioral improvements that result in it. The effects of poor self-talk become more harmful.

- **Restricted Thinking**: You say you can't do it about yourself, but the more you say that the more you accept it.

- **Perfectionism**: You often tend to accept that "fine" is not as nice as "perfect," and that quality should really be achieved. (In comparison, pure high-achievers seem to perform well than their workaholic peers, as they are usually less frustrated and satisfied with a well-functioning task instead of taking things out and cashing in on the best.

- **Depressed feelings**: Many studies have shown that poor self-talking can lead to a worsening of depression feelings. If left untreated, this may be pretty damaging.

- **Relationship Challenges**: If the relentless self-feedback makes you seem vulnerable and weak or transforming your poor self-talk into more general bad attitudes that annoy others, a loss of contact and even an "affectionate" amount of feedback will take a toll.

One of the most apparent disadvantages to negative self-talk is that it's not optimistic. It seems simple, but evidence has found that positive self-talk is a strong indicator of performance. One analysis on athletes, for example, contrasted four various forms of self-talk (educational: where sportsmen know clear tasks to do to perform well, motivational: self-talk that holds people-focused— People didn't have to learn how to do it as much as they had to tell them they're doing it fantastic and people are doing it too.

Develop Positive Self-Talk To Gain Confidence

Anyone can build constructive self-talk to gain higher self-esteem. If throughout the day you find yourself slipping into certain feelings, analyze one and work out how to bring a constructive twist on them.

A useful solution is to transform these ideas into humor. Letting yourself chuckle at criticism and throwing attention on a bad circumstance can shift your outlook a great deal. You should also seek to develop a healthy lifestyle, both mentally and physically: start healthier food and exercise three days a week, and just associate yourself with optimistic and compassionate people.

Pain stems from some pessimistic people in your community who don't trust you absolutely. So, do away with them. Trying constructive self-talk is the only step to alter harmful self-talk. This bit of advice from Mindy's aunt "The Mindy Show," Sheena — portrayed by Laverne Cox, everybody's favorite transsexual warrior from "OITNB" — ought to help:

Sheena: Ask me what you see now? Mindy: Two naked black girls in a hoody, and a big box. Sheena: It is cold. Now, if you were your best friend, the person in the mirror, would you really be as harsh and cruel to her as you are to yourself? Mindy: No! Sheena: You interact with your closest mate, and that is you!

- Flip over pessimistic thinking: Get in the routine of positive thinking by becoming more conscious of your patterns of thought. If you find a bad image, just change it. Shift to something more constructive instantly and makes you feel healthy. Dream of a beloved one, connect to an inspiring music piece, or show one of your favorite pictures.

If the pessimistic self-talk says, 'I don't know how to do that,' shift it to 'this is a perfect chance to learn anything different.' If you think you can't drop weight, adjust that to 'I'm trying to boost my health, and pursue some kind of workout I really enjoy. Optimistic thinking is a lot better than a pessimistic one. When you see the bottle partially empty, rather than half full, try to change your perspective instantly. Instead of concentrating on what's wrong with your statement, concentrate now on everything that's right that works for you.

- Become your best buddy: Only think about what you frequently tell to yourself. Now picture your best mate being asked the same terms. Imagine asking them they are unappealing, they are a loser, or they are dumb. Terrible, aren't they? If you weren't going to say anything to anyone you cherish, don't tell yourself.

The phrases we used every day impact profoundly — dialect forms our connections with people and places. The way you converse with yourself is the way you cherish yourself — your ego-talk colors your sense of self. It takes many more words to build self-confidence. Numerous studies, however, suggest that ego-talking can enhance your memory, trust, emphasis, and more. From time to time, we all battle with ego-confidence. We're failing to take charge of us as we don't believe we're worth it. Or perhaps we (misleadingly) believe self-love is egotistical. The reality is, you must place your breathing apparatus first to take control of everyone. Speaking to yourself is among the most normal and underappreciated skills that we possess. Will you make anyone else talk with you about the way you talk to yourself?

The value of the inner dialogue is critical — good phrases carry beneficial benefits. This encourages self-reflection, enhances inspiration, and binds our feelings with each other. Canadian professor, Alain Morin's study indicates there is a strong connection between a more active interaction with oneself and a stronger self-awareness and self-evaluation.

3.3 How Self-Hypnosis Helps Low Self-Esteem

Seeing our doubts regularly will definitely be a tool for enhancing self-esteem and self-confidence. Still, that's a difficult task. Staying on course is challenging, and performing it over and again, even when the subconscious is screaming at us that we'd rather not. One way to perceive it is that negative self-talk is just like addictive behavior.

We can experience the discomfort our dependency brings, we can see the impact it has on our families, and we can see it physically undermining our mental wellbeing or success at work or in social environments, or anything our conscience informs us we can't do. But we cannot resist, yet. We cannot seem to be shutting off those feelings. That is almost like the temptation the "hears" user asks them to do it again.

Hypnotherapy can become so effective for poor self-esteem since its objective is to fix the thoughts. Hypnosis allows the ego and re-learns to be a positive companion in our daily interactions. We take those unreasonable and negative thinking out and recolonize the unconscious mind with more useful data. With one target, you might conceive of hypnotherapy as mediation. Hypnosis was used for millennia to help students understand to tame their minds, find true happiness, and automatic quiet thinking. However, hypnotherapy goes one leap; further-hypnosis contributes an objective.

Here's how it functions! Our words will be instructing the mind and body to a state of increased tranquility and awareness during a hypnosis session. Our brains get to be super calm, and we have access to our psyche. We may completely circumvent the rational mind and move right to the inner ear, and speak to it directly. What is more, our minds are equally susceptible to advise while we're in a hypnotic state.

And when we hear affirmations like in this state, "you're going to have trust in all you do," they're far more prone to last. We have circumvented that crucial rational layer of suggestions, which is always so fast to meet the criteria and analyze. Now, you could think: Is that all there really is to it? And the response is brief: Yes. Yes, low self-esteem hypnosis may be extremely complex; a psychotherapist can use various strategies to motivate and restore the unconscious mind.

But whatever the method, the concept remains the same: We may introduce to the unconscious in a hypnotic state fresh, more productive and more positive knowledge. But at the

very same moment, we should strive to break the destructive ways of thought that firstly affect our ego-esteem issues.

3.4 Step-By-Step Self-Hypnosis To Boost Self-Esteem

Ten percent of American citizens suffer depression, with a 20 percent rise each year. Depression may typically be attributed to a sense of self-worth or self-esteem. It is particularly true because we reside in a highly busy and fast-paced environment where taking time for personal-examination or self-development is not granted priority. It's better to be the way people like us instead of expressing ourselves. Hypnosis is a very powerful method of addressing unconscious content.

Everyone should do self-hypnosis regularly and comfortably to remove unhealthy attitudes and habits and add constructive values-to to improve self-esteem. Hypnosis is an enhanced condition of responsiveness, suggestivity, sensitivity, tolerance to feelings, stimuli, or acts, of which the end goal is to naturally obtain a favorable reaction.

You are nearly still in a trance-like state (trance, hypnagogic state), although that becomes especially apparent as you fall asleep and awaken. See how powerful TV advertisements are, and get an understanding of how suggestivity functions and see how the news has an impact over collective opinion and practice in general. During hypnotherapy, the brain moves from the usual beta-frequency thinking / sensory-motor condition (12-20 Hz) to the lower alpha level (8-12 hertz), which becomes calmer, alert, and extended – where imagination and concepts emanate – a condition of harmony and wellbeing. This is the gateway to long lost experiences and the place where the subconscious is free for fresh programming to embrace.

You will know this condition from all of the below feelings tingling your hands, numbness or twisting in your muscles, soft feeling in floating out of your body, feeling like falling, electricity flowing through your core, heightened emotions, twitching eyelids, enhanced or reduced survival, and exhaustion (while you fall asleep).

From now on, you will never speak (or even assume) offensive words about you, either in silence or vocally. I know this isn't always easy – especially if you've had negative conditioning for a lifetime, and your self-esteem is weak. But you'll be beginning new from this minute on. Assume your mind as if it were a laptop; what you are programming in will return back. You'll gain trust and self-esteem over time by constantly loading your 'machine' with optimistic views in yourself.

Self-hypnosis is a quick means of changing negative patterns of thought. Here's a basic method of hypnosis that can bring you off to a strong start, helping you develop your self-esteem and start thinking you deserve all the wonderful life you have to give.

Hypnosis Script 1

1. Create an Aim / Objective: One part of creating how you want your life to be is enjoying yourself and possessing a high amount of self-confidence.

2. Develop A Note With The Following Features: Quick and easy to comprehend, repeatable in 5 seconds or less, using mental images that will always be productive, plausible, and precise. One way to do it is to identify a limited belief. "I'm pretty fat, and nobody loves me." You should look into circumstances where that appears to be valid and how much. Is there any evidence that it might not be true? Next, turn this into an optimistic statement: "I'm feeling good in my body, and people like me."

3. If Sitting in a Relaxed Spot or Standing, Breathe Slowly: During much of the inhalation, count from your abdomen to

7, keep for a period of 2, and then exhale whilst counting to 11. Keep on for two minutes, then restate three times. You'll note that it becomes seamless.

4. Go further into visualizing the air that travels through each of 10 parts of the body and relax. In the specified order, invest about ten seconds on each: start at the head, then move to the neck, shoulders, arms, hands, abdomen, belly, butt, feet, and legs.

5. Put the target is now. State it, make it visible, feel it as though it is really occurring.

6. Visualize it as though you had already accomplished that target. Note any emotions, particularly. If they have been pessimistic or restricting, then let them all go gently. Keep on as long as it is relaxed with this.

7. Feel grateful. Invest 15-20 sec or more feeling happy to have achieved your positive goal. How good that works rely on how genuine you may make your declaration of intent seem, becoming present as though the intended intention happened in the here and now. That's how the indigenous people monks render light. They will really feel the rainfall and giving thanks to God after heading to a higher energy location and having performed sufficient rituals to touch the Great Spirit.

Recall that emotions are the fuel that sends the subconscious into practice. Contact them, and you'll be good. You will, in either situation, become very comfortable and safe from pain and anxiety. Give it a go!

Hypnosis Script 2

1. Gently close and relax your eyelids, and take a few long, steady, rhythmic breaths. Inhale in through the nose and out in circular ventilation motion through the mouth.

2. Quiet your head as you take a slow, harmonic, and deep breath. After a couple of seconds, you start feeling focused.

3. Believe in this peaceful condition, you qualify to lead a life rich, content, and full of happiness and joy. Link with a deep conviction that the very finest existence you have has to give and know it strikes a chord in each and every cell of your body and mind.

4. Feel free to let go of any false thoughts or old training and see oneself living a healthy, successful, full life. Say to yourself, gradually and continuously, in a long, steady voice, the following phrases over and over: 'I deserve to be content, safe, wealthy, and plentiful.'

5. Truly feel as you repeat the words. Feel good and satisfied, and let those emotions get stronger as you step on and get further into it. Do this for 10–15 minutes, or if you prefer, longer.

3.5 Affirmation To Raise Self-Confidence

When you tend to say bad thoughts for yourself because you're not successful so this idea is passed on to your subconscious. Then the subconscious expresses everything that it gets. As a consequence, you'll start to run into circumstances that would disturb your trust in your skills.

When you think about yourself (even casually) in a derogatory manner, you put your own benefit in danger. The scientific stream has now established that our brain tends to produce fresh neurons during our life, which is termed neuroplasticity, the capacity to reorganize our wiring. Which means change is never too late. We should learn different talents, alter old practices, and build new ones. With new creeds, we will rewire our brains.

I shine forth and earn love and appreciation.

I respect me and acknowledge who I am.

I'll never be lonely in seeking performance. In planned and unforeseen forms, the world is helping me.

Wherever I go, I am liked and valued.

I'm self-reliant, imaginative, and ambitious with all that I do.

I feel special in my strengths and skills, so I will not accept any.

I deserve all, which is good.

I am full of caring, happy, optimistic, and productive thoughts, which eventually turn into experiences in my life.

Customers are finding merit in my work, and I am graciously compensated.

I am special, and I have unique dreams and aspirations. I do not need anybody to prove myself.

I love all the good things in my life.

I am motivated by a solution. Each issue represents an opportunity to develop.

I'm not a prisoner, and I live in the moment.

I enjoy my life to the fullest.

I'm not a Tree and have the right to alter the way I see fit.

I'm the sole responsibility for making my choices and decisions.

I'm not egoistic in placing my needs first.

I am aware of my power, and I behave with trust.

I can detect and operate on my capacity deficit.

Life is good and satisfying.

The universe blesses me with abundance, happiness, and health.

I love what I got. I believe in my passion for you.

I'm bold. My eyes represent my soul's energy.

I feel optimistic and positive. The world is conspiring to make me succeed.

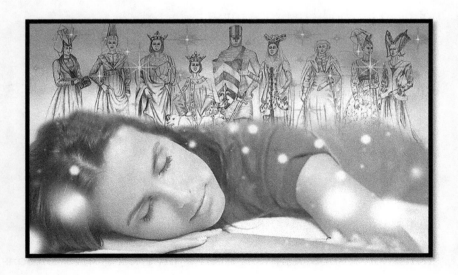

Chapter 4: Hypnosis – A Pathway To Access Past Lives

This chapter contains everything you need to know about reincarnation, past life regression therapy, and past life traumas. In the beginning, we will learn about the tell-tale signs and symptoms of a past life. These are unbreakable habits, unreasonable phobias, weird obsessions, unexplained dreams, a certain type of birthmarks, and extreme pain. But, the biggest of all is déjà vu, which we will discuss further. Then, the chapter will dive deeper into past life traumatic experiences and how they affect this current life even if we don't remember them at all. Afterward, we'll come to the topic of how to hypnosis can help with recovering past life as well as the hidden memories of our childhood. Finally, we will end the chapter with two scripts for past life regression hypnosis.

4.1 Signs Of A Past Life

We all have lived in the past. There is nothing like a "fresh spirit" For thousands of generations, all of humanity has been reborn, and in fact, no "death" remains, only that of flesh. Did you ever think where you used to exist before? Maybe you've had the impression you've traveled places before, or met anyone a long while ago - perhaps your mind tells you 'no,' but your core says 'yes.'

Many of us have encountered Deja vu at some stage in our lives. Many of us have had repeated visions of environments or individuals or events, even when there is no rational reason. I personally know of people who have developed extreme hallucinations and irrational fears of things that really don't make any sense some of them at all. Most of their life is shadowed by an irrational anxiety-until they walk into the sun. A reincarnation enthusiast also feels reassured as past lives are discovered by periods of déjà vu, visitors instantly feel comfortable with former acquaintances, and unfamiliar locations visited. These are only two of the indications that other people assume are reminders of previous lives. They are experiences concealed deep inside the pending subconscious discovery.

1. Déjà Vu

Deja Vu is that bizarre, sudden feeling that you get when you're hit by a sense that you've executed, heard, or felt it before. It can be evoked by anything from a person's face to an aroma, a taste, or attending a new place that you don't ever recollect visiting in this lifetime. Every time you get this feeling, it's a clue to the kind of past life that you may have lived. The sensation of Deja vu may be deeply disturbing as it is sometimes brief and too ambiguous to provide you specific details. Additionally, the experience of Deja vu is often prompted by a film's recollection. Or, it is induced by a connection that the present conditions have to something that's been overlooked since childhood.

2. Weird Memories

One of the more prominent indicators of past lives is distorted memories, which may appear at any moment and can be more comprehensive than those synonymous with the sensation of Deja vu. You may note, for example, that there is something odd in such memories when you compare them against others' memories and discover that there is little similarity. Of course, there's also the possibility for that to merely come down to inaccurate recollection or even to fantasy, you've had in adolescence and then interpreted as genuine. To say whether they're true memories of previous lives, search for stuff you might really find out that you couldn't think about (such as unique places, objects, or fine-grained specifics of a place).

3. Dreams and Nightmares

Experiences of past life relapse sometimes arise in your dreams, exhibiting intense hallucinations or delusions that stay with you even after you wake up. In the case of flashbacks, you can often remember traumas encountered in your previous lives, such as events that have become painful to live with and may require more processing. As with seemingly significant memories, it is important to look for minor details that may seem trivial and yet retain the essential to unlocking the life you used to live. In specific, watch for evidence of where you might have ended up living and try to notice it all you recollect when you wake up. With just a little bit of analysis, you can start to constrain your past life down to a particular country, town, or village. Often we see the same vibrant vision in minute detail, a day in and day out of deeper understanding. It may be that somebody from our families will see the same vision too! This is a common memory snapshot of past lives spent together that may be discussed in former life Regression Sessions.

4. Phobias

If talking about recalling past life events, the mind does not automatically run to the possibility of phobias! But, such apparent worries and annoyances may still be related to old encounters from former lives, so take care of them. Many phobias are very normal and, therefore, much unlikely to be connected to previous lives. In comparison, the forms of phobias that may suggest past lives involve unreasonable and very detailed concerns. Think about water, a certain number, a form, an entity, and so on. Consider that either of such concerns is related to any hallucinations or experiences you've already associated with a past life. For example, you may also fear water and frequently dream of drowning in one place.

5. Obsessions

It's good to be mindful, on a better level that previous lives can contribute to meaningful and rewarding encounters (not only worries, hallucinations, and disturbing memories!). A deep, unshakable enthusiasm that forms who you are is one of the strongest indicators of an earlier life relation. Here, we're not only talking about activities you want to do in your free time. Instead, the emphasis is on desires that you can't stop, and that sound as important to you as oxygen. There are endless instances about how these kinds of desires may manifest, but they are often innovative. So if you can't live without songwriting, can't go a day without reading, or they always save up for new supplies of painting, you may have had a related profession in your past life. And with such creative endeavors, if you can just let your imagination keep flowing, you may even see elements of your previous lives starting to emerge in your work.

6. Unbreakable Habits

We often have compulsions and behaviors that are tough to describe. However, some of these may be the result of past lived experiences. Again, as with enthusiasm, the ones you need to take more notice of are the ones you can't control. In terribly challenging cases, these habits may even become obsessions and may be problematic in everyday life. Obsessive-compulsive traits are appropriate here, although they may be mightiest. Often think about the little rituals you use to be relaxed about. For example, an item you use close by, a routine you have for relaxing, and a simple act you do to settle down. With any of these, think of what could justify them in your recent memory. If you can't locate an answer, search with connections to the patterns and the other knowledge regarding past life.

7. Severe Pain

This goes without mentioning that any chronic suffering will be carefully examined by medical practitioners. Some illnesses and disorders are challenging to identify and can involve a long-winded clinical process. Furthermore, once the clinicians have explored any potential reasons regarding a form of suffering you have; don't ignore the possibility that the distress may be related to previous lived experience. An apparent explanation here is an ache, which refers to an illness you have suffered in a former life or that you might have endured as part of operation or childbirth. Attach that discomfort to the image you are creating from your past life and note any other signs that may describe it. If, say, you still have an odd painful leg, and you often dream of running, you may have been an athlete.

8. Birthmarks

Finally, one of the main indicators and indications of visible past existence is a birthmark. All of us have one or two of these, although we sometimes merely ignore them as meaningless. They could be triggered by our place in the uterus, our birth, or natural pigment patterns. However, those who research the essence of rebirth have also questioned if such markings may be direct proof of past lives. There are two forms through which the birthmarks can be related to reincarnation. First, they can be passed down across a succession of lives, so (if prominent) they can provide you with a means to search at images of yourself through previous lives. Second, they can refer to an old life accident. You may see a pink or brown mark wherever you have been injured in one of the past lives.

4.2 Trauma and Past Life Regression Therapy (PLRT)

A psycho-spiritual type of recovery, past life regression therapy allows you to trust your imagination's strength and be willing to experience not just the pleasant, but also the grim and upsetting images of past existence. Individuals who perform psychological reconstruction of past life have advanced experience in triggering the rare condition of awareness that is required to provide something more than a snapshot of a past existence. The process really is a type of hypnotherapy. Past Life Regression is a type of hypnosis that enables the client to recall meaningful events from an unknown and unidentified past that now affects the client. In a consultation, a person may encounter a different generation, a different ethnicity, and even a separate race than they are in time at this location.

The regression of past experience is basically driven by

hypnosis. You are placed in a profoundly comfortable and alert state and informed regarding what you can see or feel; thoughts and feelings that emerge are then translated into a coherent picture of a past existence. Having been directed by this story, the workshop includes utilizing the revealed story to explain problems with your own life and how insights learned from the relapse should be adapted to them.

When you reenact a former life trauma throughout a regression, you actually get firsthand access to past life's feelings, senses, knowledge, and experience. This will contribute to an extreme, a bit of relief of suppressed thoughts and feelings, most typically anxiety, sorrow, rage, shame, or remorse. The encounter will also treat a phobia, paranoia, and psychogenic conditions such as migraines, sleep issues, severe exhaustion, trouble with the stomach, and a number of mysterious body pains.

When the problem you're grappling with in this lifespan is particularly painful and nuanced, professionally qualified professionals provide the best and most successful past life healing. An intense, cathartic response is often a necessary and valuable part of the regression of past life, and those responses are best handled by an individual trained to work with this reaction.

The PLRT procedure is a multi-step process. The therapist:

2. Guides you to access the stored memories in your subconscious

3. Helps you to make correlations between the past and the present

4. Helps you grasp and analyze the data

5. Works with you until a cure or resolution is reached

To allow you to have a more vivid experience, your hypnotherapist can ask a set of questions during PLRT.

- What do you wear? How old are you, then? What was your name?

- What is it that you see about you?

- And what's the name for the place in which you are?

- What is the time of day and date?

- What do you do, and why do you do it, or how do you feel about everything?

Is anybody there with you? Who's that, and why do they come with you? How are you feeling for this person?

Regression therapy may not be for everyone, as are many types of treatment modality. Regression of past life is often associated with rebirth. There have been reports that a conviction in the possibility of reincarnation (or at least a friendliness) is the strongest indicator of recording past life memories. On the other side, doubters or nonbelievers are considered to be less prone to record these memories.

Regression counseling in the past life is usually considered to be the strongest approach to help individuals follow a spiritual direction and its increasing acceptance as a type in therapeutic healing. But whether you practice a faith or not, it is believed that you acquire a spiritual knowledge of becoming more than a human being by knowing yourself as a spirit in certain lifetimes.

Therapists will differ in how they want to perform meetings, and how long each session would last and how much time the therapy itself will commit to the regression component. So you should anticipate your hypnotist to begin by asking you several questions regarding your current life, and the problems you want to fix. They must work together just to discover common trends that may be the source of life-long issues.

Having discussed the aspects, you are most keen to explore. You're in a greater place to search back on your past lives-this will act as the session's focus or intent. Afterward, your hypnotist will talk to you through breathing exercises steps to allow you to relax deeply. This will enable you to reach valuable latent memories-which will derive in this lifespan, or in the past, from others.

We can't say definitively as to what you would feel through regression therapy because it is done differently by all. Some individuals may catch glimpses of many past lives while others can dig through one in more depth, or uncover bad memories from their present lifetime.

How Does Past Life Trauma Manifest?

It amazes hypnotists that by constructing emotional and physical barriers to conception, anything like dying at birth two hundred years ago, will induce the spirit to make sure it won't happen again. Or the poor self-esteem, irrational anxieties, aggressive responses to certain men, trouble decision-making, and almost any fight-or-flight response are all linked to past existence.

It may be difficult to tackle past-life issues, but the benefits are immense. In reality, I don't believe you will really be the person you are supposed to be without taking your past lives into account.

Below is some of the interesting aspects in which past lives show themselves:

Constipation: Bleeding out at the conclusion of a lifetime can give rise to fear of losing power. Another indication that constipation is a past-life problem is that when you move, it gets worse and then recovers as you discover the source of the initial past-life.

Water: Bringing a ship down induces distrust of water. Not normally a concern in a pool, but the sight of warm, dark water will cause fear.

Writer's Block: Usually the block is a fear of rejection (what if people don't like me or my writing?), a fear of self-expression (what if it comes back and bites me?), a fear of judgment (what would people think of me?) and a fear of inferiority (whom should I consider myself a writer?). All of which, you got it, originates from a previous lifespan.

Poverty: Moving from a life of fair comfort to being impoverished in a past life may turn out to be a fear of being a lady bag, a desire to put away wealth, or the feeling that almost everything you have or have worked for maybe stripped away from you.

Sleep issues: Horrific experiences thousands of years ago during the dark hours will trigger the mind to go on high alert when it is expected to sleep. Do you start waking up at a given time every night or most? Your soul is worried that history tends to repeat itself, so it needs to wake you up to check that all is well.

Indecision: If you were in charge of making a decision that helped cause your demise or the demise of someone else, then you might find it difficult to choose between two minor matters, such as ordering pasta or fish on a menu. Your spirit will despise to be held responsible even for the tiniest decision - making.

Past-life trauma discloses itself in so many ways! If it's an aversion of close clothes (restraint in a dungeon), a fear to hiking (a jail in slave camp), or cold extremities (dying from frostbite), almost two decades in my practice as a real-life medium shows me that the trigger is still in the real. On a more optimistic side, past lifespans as a pastry chef in this lifetime should allow the dough to work with you. As a singer, several renditions can help you pull a melody out of certain instruments. And numerous lives in outdoor activities will give you peace of mind as a warrior. It is not only the pain of past lives that persists with us but the gifts that we have built over several incarnations. The kid savants you see across the web are a perfect illustration, including the 5-year-old acting as though she'd been practicing for centuries. (Naturally, she does, but just not in this life.)

Since learning what occurred to your spirit before this single rebirth helps you to overcome the doubts and other obstacles and draw on the gifts, you have built over the years more efficiently.

The closest you get to fulfill the life your parents wanted, the better you appreciate your past lives and take the actions you need to recover from their impact. And who wouldn't like to live a better, satisfying life?

4.3 Recovering Hidden Memories with Hypnosis

The most famous memories of previous lives are what you are unintentionally mindful of, as those details are very quietly exposed. For instance, unique dislikes that have no foundation in your present life could be either from an incident in your past life or a negative attachment to that incident. Such a response, physical or emotional, will also leave you baffled because there is no rational explanation for this deep aversion. Fears and phobias are among the most typical residuals of an earlier life case. These latent memories sometimes seem erratic and without any rhyme or meaning, but once you start delving into your previous lives, you may uncover the explanation behind unexplained personal preferences and dislikes.

Have any of you ever first met somebody, but had an unexplained hostile attitude to that individual? You might have feared the individual, or you may have had an extreme hatred for the person, and yet there is no rational answer for such a powerful negative response. Like the lady's reaction to lemon drops, a previous-life negative association can carry over into a traumatic memory.

There have been two think tanks around cellular recollection. Both assume memories are stored inside your cells.

- Ancestral Memories

The first hypothesis of cellular memory notes that what is considered to be past life recollection are simply memories of the ancestors. The human taps into the cellular memories preserved in the inherited form. Such experiences are transferred down the generations. A good illustration sometimes given is how dogs innately learn how to herd goats or cattle from a long series of herding puppies. It is theorized

that the empathic recollections of ancestors integrated inside the genetic code may be taped into.

- Personal Cellular Memories

The second leading explanation theorizes that an individual carries its experiences through cellular memory from one lifetime to another. The spirit itself is a mixture of energy-life. It imprints certain experiences on the body at the moment the soul reaches the different body, also at the time of conception. This hypothesis is also used to describe physical differences between people that attribute different personalities from past lives. If the mind is the manifestation of these strong forces, then the mind is the source of all perceptions in creation. That means the person will tap into certain memories by triggering certain cells. Several hypotheses extend to involve the concept that certain cells are released over time with different desires, instincts, and thoughts to lead the person for their current embodiment in its true course.

Indeed hypnosis has the potential to boost memory. It does this mainly by strengthening the processes by which we produce the aforementioned memories and simply repeat them. It again largely depends on your suggestivity and reasonableness. These two can be used before the required

piece of knowledge is produced to facilitate intensified analysis.

Memory retrieval hypnosis will help you discover secret experiences that may be out of control of your usual waking state. The tension of it will drive your memory much farther away when you miss anything significant. There's no excuse to sit confused because of cognitive issues. A professionally qualified hypnotist on memory rehabilitation will help you activate the memories. We may probably have such unobservant times. You have all experienced the scenario where in the middle of a conversation; you just couldn't immediately recall addressing a question. You know the right answer, but at that point in time, for some rationale, you just can't remember. You might also know the letter in which the response ends, but yet it just rests on the tip of the tongue.

Although this can be annoying and disturbing, it's relatively common. It might not be a huge deal because it's something easy and boring that has been overlooked, but when it's something that impacts your existence and prevents your development, it's crucial to get support from outside. Hypnosis and meditation include hypnosis for cognitive restoration and enable you to recover exposure to certain

experiences that have been lost and obscured.

Maybe you wrote the key on a slip of paper to your safe and tucked it inside, and now you can't locate it, or maybe you've got a work trip planned, so you just aren't able to recall where you put your passport. The more upset you feel over the scenario, the more complicated it would be to remember information.

Regenerating memory will help you unlock those gates behind which the experiences are concealed. The hypnotist of memory restoration can softly lead you into a calm environment that liberates you from pressures and helps you to concentrate on the unconscious places where certain secret experiences are kept. Not only does this higher level of consciousness encourage you to view certain memories, but it also helps you to remember what prompted them to disappear away. Sometimes as trauma happens, certain thoughts are kept locked away from a conscious mind. This process is a self-protection tool, but it can be a major hindrance at times too. However, if the waking mind is not available to memory, the incident often influences how you perceive and how you react to incidents in life. If you notice that some events trigger a powerful emotional response but don't recall previous interactions that could have contributed to certain reactions, maybe memory hypnosis may support you.

You no more have to remain a reluctant hostage to certain feelings with the aid of a professional memory recovery hypnotist, and no one will press the buttons anymore. Healing from childhood violence and perhaps other trauma may improve.

Many of the advantages of memory restoration hypnosis include:

- Better Recall

- Feeling relieved

- The better feeling of stillness

- Putting away worries and irrational fears

- The self-esteem improved

- External disputes settled

- Better control of your emotions

A memory rehabilitation session usually requires about one to two hours completing from start to finish. Therapists talk about what ushered you here, what you'd like to achieve. It's important to communicate any details you remember so that the hypnotist can better guide you effectively. Your hypnotist, with a controlled message, will help you calm your body and ease your mind through hypnosis.

The hypnotist would also ask you questions and make you retrace previous experiences so you can continue processing images removed from your consciousness. This journey exposes the forgotten memories and allows you to see them from a new viewpoint, so you can fix them and make progress. It's advised that you seek to rebuild your memories yourself as far as practicable in case you have forgotten anything. It is only after you have failed to recreate the recollection that you can now call in a hypnotist.

Ultimately, the influence of hypnotherapy is often experienced through the human brain's activities. Through entering a trance, you encourage the hypnotist to direct you more profoundly into the conscious and subconscious sections of your mind. Such pieces are beyond the scope of the alertness process in ordinary circumstances. Therefore it provides unimpeded entry to the inner parts of the human mind's network.

Broadly speaking, we rarely have experiences fully lost or overlooked absolutely. Nevertheless, we cannot even recall a large chunk of such processed knowledge without taking additional effort to recover it. We can't only discount the strength and importance of hypnotherapy for any purpose.

4.4 Deep Sleep Hypnosis for Past Life Recall

Almost always, past-life recollections are discovered by using hypnotic regression, meaning you are placed into a "hypnotic" or extremely comfortable state, and then "repressed" (moved backward) to an earlier time.

Here is a script for guided hypnosis for past-life recall.

Script 1

"I'll pick up your right hand in a moment and count to 3, and drop it down. When it comes to rest, in time, you take trips backward in time. You grow younger, returning to your birth date and start to fly back in time before you move through a particular lifespan. "(Repeat 2 to 3 times.)

"Ready now 1, 2, and 3"

(Dropping the hand) "You fly back through time – becoming younger and younger – back to the early days you were raised. Continue to travel backward in time till you come into another lifetime.

(Pause for about 3 seconds, and then press the front of your client.) Is it daylight or night - time? Where are you? "(Get a reply) Are you in or out?"

Explore each scene, and move as appropriate to the next one.

Ending meeting with "I'll proceed between one and five in a second. On number five, return to the office (or from wherever you started) eyes closed and relaxed deeply."

Script 2

Let's begin by slowly counting one to ten. You are growing ever more with each number

Okay, be relaxed.

One… Your eyes are calming, and if you like, you should shut them.

Two…. Your body becomes loosened, unstrung from your feet.

Three…. Relax your toes.

Four…. Relax your legs and torso.

Five…. Relaxing thorax, neck, head, body, legs, fingertips

Six…. Relax your arms, your back, your hands, your chin, your teeth, your nose, and your eyes.

Seven…. Your head's crown lightens and softens muscles.

Eight.... Your entire body is slackening.

Nine.... You experience a sense of warmth, lightness, and drifting.

Ten.... You are in a state of trance.

Eleven.... You feel happy, confident, and healthy.

I welcome you to walk into a safe and pleasant climate. This may be a forest, greenhouse, pasture, shore, hillside, anywhere you know, or anywhere you. Witness the attractions, the sounds, the smells, the emotions, flavor if necessary.

You will come on a path, wandering through your scene, and you can follow that if you like the path. With each further step that you take, it takes you to greater depth into a trance. The sounds and the colors take you deeper, etc.

Feel a vivid, a more friendly scent, hear a more relaxed sound. This is the scene of your fantasies.

Yeah, you should tell me whatever you're going through and how you look when you go deeper into your own hidden woods.

You will want to visit this monastery while you are able where you will explore your history.

You will find a long sloping hall of mirrors after joining it, they have the foundation.

Looked small on the outside, you might find it's vast on the inside. You will look at the mirrors.

Some mirrors are in mahogany color, others of them in white or other fabrics. May be any mirrors are even ornamented, some simple, others embellished or crafted cases. There may well be any mirrors that are oval, triangular in some forms, and circular in others.

The reflective space, maybe in a spiral around the temple, appears to roll on forever.

Looking into such reflectors, you could see variants of yourself at various ages in your existence.

You may also see yourself from your youth, or teen years, in a common mirror.

And yet again, you will see older copies of yourself as you proceed down the sloping hallway.

You've seen the way you looked in many lifetimes. You may feel attracted to one special mirror. You can contact him/her when you're ready. The mirrors will give you a good picture, a dream of yourself on a particular day.

The mirror transforms into a soft nebula, and like Alice in Through the Looking Glass, you may want to travel over the gleaming floor. You can see it on the opposite side of that wall recognizing that the positive energy is starting to act as protector and guides you. When you explore your history, you can experience a sense of time changing. Get it

When you're ready, you'll be directed securely back to reality.

I encourage you to head right and gaze at yourself from the hand in the reflection. Can you tell us what your gender is? Which race? What era? What type and sort of body?

Can you note any visible identifying features? What do you wear?

Now take a look down and see your feet. Are you barefoot or wearing shoes? What does the ground seem like?

Understand that the reflection portal stays where this is (like the Narnia lamp post) and is easy to access.

Know when you're good for traveling. Now you might want to switch into this new atmosphere and want to explore.

Let's move forward in this past lifetime towards your death. Know you are a human being

Getting a subjective consciousness and moving in all-time into or out of various life forms.

Death is something not to be scared of; it is merely a bridge to life and the inter-life of life.

The Higher, Immortal Self, as always, will be around to direct you through such a journey.

Where did you die this time in your life? So what are your experiences of the phase?

After you moved through that process, were you changed?

See now your soul in the Inter-life, the peaceful and soothing place between us.

What do you think? What is your impression of this place? Are they accustomed? Would you like to

Would you know anybody out there with you?

The Inter-life will be a way to rewrite and repair our lives.

I may add, if appropriate: It is a unique spot to cure life traumas, study what we've experienced and what we're not discovering.

You're actually between entire lives, remembering your reflected copies.

Gently shift from who you were previously and who you are today.

What learning have you learned from the past? What skills should be learned?

Are you enjoying your real life? Would you remember someone in your daily existence from this entire previous life?

Are there some questions only now being sorted out?

If the individual you have been from the other existence could communicate to you what he or she will have to tell you? What do you have to do to carry past and current healing? Will you have any?

Is this past life resonant with your current life?

Simply say it whenever you feel ready, and I would help you back to a condition of maximum consciousness.

Now is the time to start moving back to the maximum focus of the outer world, living in the present.

Remember that there is still that which is kept inside. You'll notice that you know all of this.

This journey has taken place, and you might find that far more information is coming to you so that you do

Process and incorporate knowledge to help you in continuing your development and wholeness.

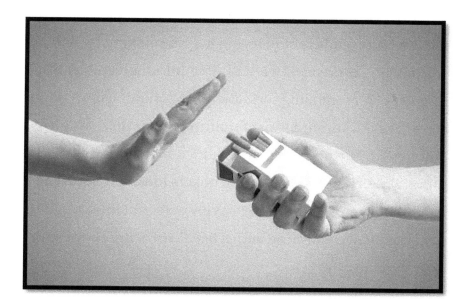

Chapter 5: Deep Sleep Hypnosis – An Effective Method To Quit Smoking

This chapter will begin by introducing the power of the subconscious mind and why it is vital in trying to quit any kind of addiction but particularly smoking. Then, we'll move on to the limitations inherent in trying to quit smoking by only using willpower. Afterward, we will dive into the benefits of Sleep hypnosis for smoking cessation and how using the subconscious is a surefire way of quitting rather than simply using willpower. Furthermore, the chapter will then discuss some mindfulness tips and tricks all smokers looking to quit can use. After that, there will be a sleep-hypnosis script towards the end. And finally, we will close with a list of affirmations for smokers who looks to quit.

5.1 Subconscious Mind - The Root Of All Addictions

The majority of smokers get stuck on a daily ritual they despise. That is accurate. Most smokers- an estimated 80%-would be happy never again to smoke a further cigarette.

It does make much sense too. We all realize a cigarette is detrimental to your well-being. Also, mild smokers felt a throat infection or breathing trouble when they ascended a set of stairs. And, of course, there is the danger of more serious consequences on health. (Tobacco is responsible for hundreds of thousands of deaths per annum worldwide, as per the World Health Organization.)

There are zillions of other justifications to quit, not mentioning, saving money, getting beautiful skin for your children, being more productive, etc. But if most people who smoke want to discontinue, have lots of reasons to stopped smoking, and understand just how harmful cigarettes are to their well-being, what keeps them from doing so?

The possible explanation for that is straightforward. Nicotine dependency is ingrained deeply in the sub-consciousness. Stress, mealtime, walking, smoking (and the list just goes on) all subconscious levels cause nicotine cravings. But what if your head had a way of "shutting off" that voice? Or at best re-frame the implicit thinking to talk about cigarettes negatively? The user will start untangling and quiet the network of subconscious emotions that hold the problem in place with the aid of a hypnotherapist or through self-hypnosis.

Nicotine abuse is a barrier to the conscience. Because of physical and mental addiction, nicotine is such a hard habit to kick. Active compulsion, which may trigger signs of withdrawal, serves as a roadblock to leave.

Following are the common symptoms of nicotine withdrawal:

- Lethargy

- Irritability

- Pains and aches

- Pain in the chest

- Migraines

Yet while the symptoms of nicotine withdrawal are painful, something is occurring at a deeper level, which makes it so difficult to stop smoking. Our subconscious minds sustain an addiction to nicotine. During supper, or when you do get behind the throttle, the unconscious causes the desire for a smoke. It's the subconscious mind that causes a pang when you're under tension or get a bottle of wine dumped into it. This internal struggle also illustrates why most smoking quitting supports are largely unsuccessful, such as nicotine replacement. Only physical cravings are removed by NRT – but those mental impulses, those subconscious impulses which tell us to grab for a cigarette, are very much in existence. But curing tobacco abuse needs addicts to fight them head-on emotional war. Due to the top-down processing of the mind, the battle continues in your subconscious.

Assume an addict who wants to leave needs a major briefing on the work. She is definitely feeling stressed out. The use of a cigarette could then trigger stress. But from where do all these signals originate? The top-down analysis may be effective in understanding the process.

All the sensory input we receive is being sent to the subconscious in a nutshell-touch, scent, thoughts, and sights. The unprocessed sensory data is transported to the nervous system, where it creates a conscious perception. The brain here defines thoughts and perceptions and produces an answer. In other terms, the mind absorbs the signal of tension, worries of what is going on, and then generates a reaction that is focused on such thoughts. It is that phase that makes it extremely hard to quit smoking. Subconscious emotions are shaping our reactions from the top down. You may equate cigarettes as a way to relax, for example, and so your normal reaction to stress may be to illuminate. The trick to stopping smoking is to obtain top-down power-suppressing the unconscious reinforcement reaction that holds the dependency in place.

Simply because you decide to leave doesn't necessarily mean you will. Have you ever questioned why traditional reduction of smoking therapies such as patches of nicotine, nicotine gums, and pharmaceutical drugs perform so poorly? While they can reduce your nicotine cravings, the temptation to "light up a cigarette" may always prevail. Since your subconscious has been so addicted to it through the many years of addiction, it actually requires the "ritual" of addiction. Here is where the subconscious gets into play

If you didn't realize, much of your mind's subconscious component makes up, probably about 90% of your consciousness. And if that's not enough, then here is where the mind's main processing takes place. In your subconscious, there are both the convictions, emotions, and the origin of the compulsive behaviors. And, unfortunately, with those belief systems or thinking, you cannot interfere.

Here is an instance. Let's assume you're horribly frightened of dogs because when you were a kid, you were bitten by one. The hatred of dogs was practically burned into the subconscious mind on that day. No matter, however hard I want to reassure you of my sweet Rottweiler's cuteness, you will always be scared by it. The same holds valid about smoking, but it is a disease that has burnt itself "slowly" into the subconscious. That is the reason why it's so easy to just say something like "Hey, I'm not going to smoke from next week on." It would be my last cigar ever, I promise," I say. Okay, the brain thinks differently. But don't abandon heart, maybe someone can tell him that smoking is bad.

5.2 Why Willpower Is Not Enough When Quitting

The temptation to smoke depends on the urge to light a cigarette, and not the other way around! Adjust the way you think and the way you feel regarding cigarettes, and you'll be a non-smoker now. Nicotine performs a trick on our minds, causing smokers to think the cigarette allows them to sleep, deal with depression, or remain slim. Still, isn't that true? If that is real, then ALL addicts on this world will be happy, calm, and clearly the skinniest community of men. And why do addicts tend to smoke even though they think they intend to discontinue?

Trying to give up smoking while actually believing that a cigarette is an explanation of why you can relax, deal with stress, and refrain from instilling cravings in food is like telling a rope to push water, which is almost unrealistic.

Imagine not attempting to ponder a red kitty, a red kitty in a red tree. What have you ever conjured up in your imagination- a red cat in a red forest, right? That is just how to tell oneself not to have smoke. Whenever you think you do not have a cigarette, you believe you want to have a cigarette. Sounds resonant? Absolute determination is no substitute for the internal struggles occurring inside an addict's brain.

The medication nicotine isn't your friend, but it's just one of the excuses you can't stay off the cheery-go-round. Did you both sleep all night? Then during this time, you were a non-smoker, not even dreaming about tobacco. Wouldn't it be good not to worry about the next smoke, to enjoy your life? What, instead, would an addict do?

Smokers are fully conscious of the safety hazards and smoking costs, but they often smoke. It is the moral structure of a smoker that produces the will to consume. If the biases are revealed and modified, it is easier to overcome the practice of cigarettes. If you truly think there's nothing to surrender, that is when you are the non-smoker. The transition is complete without desires, with no signs of withdrawal, or weight gain. Within two days, you'll be fully drug-free but feel great instantly.

Why do people who stop go back to cigarettes? It's because they didn't use multiple methods & strategies to deal with the pressures of life. By learning and incorporating new physical, mental, and nutritional techniques, a person can remain free from smoke for the rest of their lives.

For years now, the idea that people suffering from smoking or substance abuse are actually missing moral strength has transcended culture. Those who have suffered have been seen as flawed, morally corrupt, and missing the strength to regulate their own behavior. Luckily, both scientific knowledge, as well as the medical profession, has begun to regard alcohol addiction and substance abuse as an illness — and not an inability of power or strength of will. Research studies are a tremendous benefit in explaining the fact that dependency is actually a disorder and not just a matter of possessing low will strength. The review concluded with the following facts:

1. Reward pathways in the brain are numbed, which makes it difficult for individuals to feel pleasure or gain an incentive to complete daily activities

2. Progressively primed reactions to drug abuse, implying the ability to overcome cravings is gradually getting worse.

3. The weakening of regions of the brain involved in decision-making, inhibition control, and self-regulation, making chronic recurrence highly likely. Most of the people who have discovered long-term sobriety can attest to firm resolutions to never drink/use in our past again. For stretches of time, we may also have succeeded in "white-knuckling" it. However, as for those battling depression and/or abuse, only having a solid commitment to leave never suffices.

The truth is that we need action to move ahead on our resolution, such as seeking help. While this does not happen easily to many people, if we expect to achieve long-term, worthwhile normalcy, it is absolutely essential for a large percentage of us to.

"Of course," you think you'd like to quit, but if you search deep enough, you'll discover a part of you comparable to or better than your desire to stop smoking. Isn't it an actuality that we're all in power and that in most aspects of life, we can do what we desire? Needless to say! And why is it you have always not started smoking. The strength of hypnotherapy lies in that. Because you really do not want to quit smoking in your unconscious or subconscious mind! So you are really in power; you are just deciding not to quit yet on some other state of consciousness. When there is a thought or routine of contradiction in your unconscious or sentimental mind, it overrides all ambition in your reasonable or conscious mind toward success. Feelings would always win when the feelings and reasoning are in confrontation.

You can say to yourself, "I know I want to stop smoking," then at the same moment you hear voices inside you saying, "But I would want to smoke!" So a good quote is," What we say not always what we experience, but what we experience is what is going on in our lives. We frequently hear such a statement, I know I'm all right, but feel insufficient. I know I look really good, but I don't feel beautiful, I know I've got enough money but I feel like I don't! "These sorts of arguments are the explanations we're often not successful when our subconscious mind has a contradiction. In our sub-consciousness the notifications are like the software on the hard drive of our machine. They were written or embedded for our bio-computer to run. It's not always what we see on the screen that will be written in our memory. The conscious mind is the projector, and our hard disk is unconscious.

The hard drive was established when we stopped smoking several years earlier. Cigarettes were presented as though they were perfect. They left us feeling comfortable. They have helped us cope with life problems, and perhaps even made us seem more appealing. Today the subconscious is using old signals to operate life. Observe anytime you hear a single being performed on the radio that was famous with your first love when you were 16. You'll automatically begin to recall all of the memories of that period. Not only do you talk about the time, but you'll also begin to experience the feelings of that moment. You can remember what you wear, who you were with, and what the climate that day was like. You also might remember the last advert about cigarettes on TV that was in 1970. Time stands still to the subconscious mind.

That is an anchor. It means a perceived recollection. Another definition of an anchor is the scent of a fragrance that was essential to you in life at a younger period. It might be your mom's perfume or smell cooking dinner while you were pretty young or your grandma baking bread for you. You will be there practically as if it were yesterday. I encourage you when the sensation occurs, not to remember certain memories. That is almost unlikely. The music is playing, and without any thinking, the mind moves through that moment. It is exactly what occurs when you speak about a cigarette. During traffic jams, you light up, an instant of anxiety you light up after dinner, start celebrating, and a cigarette is wanted! These and other stimulation will introduce back the memory of a period when a cigarette was essential in life at an earlier time. I defy you not to think of smoke when that stimulus takes place.

The power of such a type of memory goes further than our conscious awareness. Conscious experience is when you think you don't smoke, and then the unconscious thought does the opposite. If I suggest you not to think about an elephant, what do you think of it? Very definitely an elephant! This is named "Reverse-effect Law!" It means the stronger you try to prevent you from getting. That is what happens when you decide to stop marijuana, too. What you can think of here is a cigarette. The more necessary it is not to carry it to the surface, the further the subconscious does. If I say that not thinking about an elephant is worth $5 million, the need for doing the reverse gets much stronger. If you're advised you're going to risk your work status if you don't stop smoking or your well-being is compromised, the desire for smoking is growing much stronger.

5.3 How Hypnosis Works For Smoking Cessation

One hypothesis on why hypnosis succeeds with addiction to nicotine: it allows us the opportunity to re-frame our top-down vision. When you encounter triggers that may induce a hunger, the mind has memories already in a position that affect the reaction. You sound worn out. The anxiety activates thinking about cigarettes as a way to unwind, and you are reacting. Yet hypnosis lets you get to a state of mind where you change the mechanisms of pessimistic thought. How? Well, you follow relaxation and breathe control during hypnosis to attain a trance-like state. This state of mind is close to fantasizing; you are conscious, but the mind is detached at the very same time.

Whilst the subconscious is far more accessible to ideas in the trance-like state, it's disconnected from the vital, aware mind – the portion of the mind that is actively trying to remain a smoker for motives. Hence, a hypnotist will give you more constructive advice to "stay." In other terms, you are putting up obstacles for the passive, top-down mechanisms that keep the problem in place. And when you feel a smoking stimulus, the mind doesn't respond immediately – it slows down to "listen" to this new knowledge that you've received.

Our unconscious thinking is mighty and shapes our beliefs. And when our unconscious informs us that this should work, we bring the knowledge back down by top-down analysis. Hypnotherapy operates in similar ways. We add fresh, more detailed knowledge of smoking to our minds. Hypnotic ideas – when offered when in the state of trance – may reflect on how patterns become unconscious reactions to stimuli, and how we have the full influence of our emotions. And you could get ideas that re-frame the scent of tobacco smoke, i.e., it smells like plastic burning. Furthermore, one of the more common smoking reduction hypnosis methods is called the Spiegel's System. One of the very first psychologists to popularize therapeutic hypnotherapy, Herbert Spiegel, was the founder of "Trance and Treatment: Practical Applications of Hypnosis." Spiegel will have three recurring recommendations in a hypnotherapy outline during the sessions, including:

- Smoking is toxic

- I respect and protect your body

- You want your internal organs to live

Spiegel's system, in other terms, has not centered on talking about stopping smoking. Instead, he hypothesized that having patients concentrate on honoring the body was distracting the focus away from cessation and completely ignoring it.

Whenever it comes to addictions, hypnosis works well. Essentially, what occurs through hypnosis is that the consciousness may reach a condition known as the hypnotic trance, and in that phase, the hypnotherapist's ideas may pass peacefully into the subconscious. Expect stuff like "Cigarettes should taste like diesel gas from now on," etc. He will even make you echo the things he means, including "from this day forward I do not kill myself with smoke." Believe it or not, after a single therapy session, many individuals encounter positive results!

Hypnosis is a soothing and very fun activity when coupled with other methods, and it can feel like a child's play to put down cigarettes for good. So be not scared, too! You'll be 100 percent conscious of what's going around you through hypnosis, so be confident that the hypnotist can't force you to do some crazy stuff you don't want to do. Even if you want to see what hypnosis session sounds like, search out those YouTube videos to see for yourselves. And oh, don't worry. With the help of an amazing modality like hypnotherapy, you can stop smoking.

And what do we do when we're out of reach to such a wide extent? If you're attempting to stop, the more you want cigarettes, like how do you leave? This problem has a response, and it is pretty simple. Learn to enter the internal part of the mind where the entire pattern resides, not the external, helpless part. I gave some great examples of how mighty your unconscious mind can be. It is said that mentality can make or break us. If we look at the subconscious as a musical instrument, then we will learn to manage it with enough practice like we will be a good player. We will know how to transform our attention into a better position in life. Instead of killing it, we should encourage our inner self to enhance our well-being by smoking or bringing up certain life practices that are not beneficial to us. Even health can be improved through learning to communicate with one's inner mind. Did you ever wonder where the disease originated? It originates from the lack of comfort. We are in disquiet when we're not at comfort!

The solution to all of the concerns arrives right now. We can communicate a different message to our sub-consciousness by learning to loosen up internally. Not only take things easy and relax but also learn to go into our inner mind while we ease the outer mind because only and only then should we be able to meet life's patterns at heart and eradicate or redirect them. This will happen in a variety of ways. Some may opt for meditation or therapy or bio-feedback or hypnosis of themselves. These all have a way to reach the subconscious mind. The ability is; how we are using those techniques. Anyone will learn to play a song on the piano, just like the guitar. Playing it well will take some practice and talent, though. It is your consciousness, after all. You can learn better than anyone to redirect it. You have the power, and it's in your head.

If we believe hard enough, our inner mind listens to us? It will most likely do so, and then we will achieve our goal. If we use hypnosis to silence the outside that always seems to be trying to think of many thought processes at the same time, we can communicate directly to the inner mind. That is definitely true. To me, self-hypnosis is the most effective means of accessing the subconscious. It is like a direct link to the re-writing of messages that no longer fit our lives. You can really interact and alter an addiction quickly with hypnosis. That doesn't mean the problem can never restart, but self-hypnosis will offer us the freedom and start utilizing our logical mind and maintain the progress. The reason for this success is that by communicating to the inner mind, you're not trying to resist your own objectives. You will often think of a target and disprove that target as you say to yourself. You can tell yourself you want to give up smoking, and tell yourself at the same time that you question if you can. Or that you'll more definitely gain the weight back if you leave, so why continue. Maybe you're telling yourself you've tried a lot of times, and always go back or fail, so it's useless. Every time you want to alter the old post, you seem to have a justification for why it isn't going to fit. I'm even theorizing the old narrative is gaining strength as you keep telling yourself to give up. We have been told that we can do something by being optimistic. The obstacle is that positive thinking is at odds with subconscious training. Even if we can tell ourselves numerous times that the phrases often go unheeded to quit smoking. Perhaps a member of the family or relative asks you to give up smoking, and you get annoyed because even if you think they're right, they've made a comment. You may even be pressed as they make a comment.

5.4 Mindfulness Techniques For Smoking

One of the simple aspects about this method of mind control — what helps it function so effective in learning how to improve your patterns — is that you get out of the head and see yourself as you would like to be — from an outsider perspective (as defined in this exercise in emotional flexibility). That may sound easy, and you could think, 'Okay, what's the major deal? "So what – if you're 'stepping back' and looking at yourself the way you like to be. Why does it make a difference? 'But when you're doing the tactic in a very particular manner, in a very Conscious way, you can make that picture — that cognitive picture of yourself — so captivating that it tends to attract you, and you are drawn like a magnet away from the old behaviors and into a new life as a kind of individual freedom from that old pattern. That is, you are the sort of person you would like to be in your life, beginning now.

The system works well because, from the point of view of an observer, you can detach and see oneself in your fantasy in a new and innovative way. This little process has power and magic, and I'll demonstrate to you how to do it. The key to this NLP mind power technique, developed by one of the NLP's original founders, Richard Bandler, is imagination, visualization, and repetition. Because your subconscious is unaware of what is factual and what is fictitious, mindfulness practice and repetition can form a new habit. Most elite athletes and performers are now using internal rehearsals to enhance their results. Mental imagery is crucial to understanding how to change your behavior without repeating the new pattern again and again, physically.

In the following phase, a particular signal or stimulus is correlated with new behavior. The cue may be an object, like a mobile device, a thought, or an emotion.

By affiliating the cue repeatedly with the new experience or behavior patterns, you will generate a compulsive reaction that will be provoked whenever there is a cue or anchor.

1. Recognize your unwelcome behavior, emotion, and/or disposition.

2. What is a particular cue often present before the inappropriate behavior? It could be an image inside your head, a metaphor, or an expression.

3. See a picture of the cue a little before the undesirable behaviors and set that picture aside for a minute.

4. How can you appear like you still have a new development? You'll find that image of yourself very appealing as you make a massive, shiny colorful image of yourself already possessing this behavior change. You can see

that behavior has changed because you realize that "other you" posture. You will see a glow in his / her eyes and a comfortable grin on his / her lips while gazing at the other you are heart. You tell the other one regarding the transition, and you feel very happy, and you can sense his / her internal conversation. What precisely does he/she say?

5. See how appealing and satisfying the other you are. You do not know whether you want to become the other you, yet— the attractive one over there.

6. Is there any piece of you who disagree with this picture? If yes, adjust the image in such a way that it rectifies your criticisms until it appeals.

7. Reduce that photo now. Make it smaller and littler, and it will become a small dot.

8. Place the dot the includes the other you who already has the new action in the middle of the cue picture you previously placed (Step 2)

9. Now the two pictures, the cue picture, and the dot, swiftly exchange.

10. The cue pictured lacks brightness and gets smaller until it blends into space. The fresh you are blossoming right before you, stronger, larger, clearer, painting out your dream.

11. Now the scene empties out. The computer also shows persistent distortion.

12. Repeat with the faster process. Note the mark, which is the fresh you in the trigger picture of what you see right before the unwelcome behavior. The dot spreads, and the currency you are right in front of you, vivid and vibrant, as the background of the cue vanishes.

13. See a broad screen.

14. Then do it again quickly. With the fresh, you within you see the signal and the tiny mark. The new picture is vivid and vibrant.

15. Can you tell your telephone number backward?

16. And again! Quicker! Also, see the trigger.

17. Fuzz panel sticks.

18. Yet again. Also, see the trigger.

19. Can you reverse spell your name?

20. Quicker! See the trigger.

21. Screen blank.

22. See the cue.

23. See the broad screen.

Repeat five more times in the last two stages, faster. And then five more times, quicker still.

5.5 Sleep Hypnosis For Smoking Cessation

You can break bad habits, and come out with new automatic behaviors that best serve you by using methods of self-hypnosis to reskill your nervous system to react differently to impulses that set off the unhealthy habit. So, for example, if you're looking for a quit smoking hypnosis, your smoking triggers may include your first-morning cup of coffee, a certain time of day when you're having a cigarette break, or a feeling of anxiety or annoyance.

You will "anchor" a new reaction to certain things (or triggers) by utilizing hypnosis or self-hypnosis smoking strategies such that the reactive urge changes from a nicotine appetite to another one. Anyone who uses self-hypnosis to suggest smoking abstinence has already conquered "half the fight," which is because one of the keys to self-hypnosis performance is motivation. As a famous New York therapist says, "In hypnosis, you don't have to 'believe' to work, you just got to be willing to go through the process." And there is a big indicator of how self-hypnosis works. Your will is an unconscious guideline. When we calm down our loud, active minds, we will bring about improvements in our attitudes and responses.

So, what process do you need to be inclined to go through to give up smoking for free? Or it can be any chronic compulsive behaviors for that subject.) It's a very delicate and pleasant one, but you've got to practice it every day to get significant results. Self-hypnosis to quit drinking starts with you, perfecting the capabilities to attain a relaxing state. How really bad could this be?

This may be achieved by guided breathing, incremental calming, or mindfulness. Once you get excellent at soothing your mind and body, with self-hypnosis, you can cause a change in your habits. You will instantly eradicate a problem such as smoking by getting hypnotized and then trying to self-hypnosis to strengthen the hypnosis. Hypnotherapy is supposed to avoid cigarettes. It's up to you to stop that. I find that hypnotherapy is useful for suppressing the cravings, triggers, and smoking experiences. If you can suppress those addictions, then you'll be effective in eliminating the smoke from your existence with your initial aware inspiration.

When you want to deliberately stop cigars, the choice is up to you. Let's say that through hypnosis, all I've taught you regarding the effectiveness of smoking abstinence is open to you. Let's say it's going to be quick, you're not going to replace, and you're not going to have extreme retirements. You'd be inspired to leave, then? This is what's required to be effective. If the impulses are suppressed you deliberately plan to stop. It's our contract. You use hypnotherapy to deal with the problems you might have faced in the past and without the normal struggles, the hypnosis would bring you gliding to achievement. There is no question that hypnosis can work in suppressing the impulses, because hypnotherapy mitigates the inner control or training that used to occur. It does so by quieting from thought processes the external mind and then relaxing the internal world and allowing for current programming. It's sort of like the machine asking you to remove all software so you can load a new one. Silence the external mind so you will then rewire the internal world. It is fast!

A few directives that will enable this method to exist are to be followed. Your intention is vitally important to quit. In hypnosis, there is a common expression that means, "You can't mesmerize somebody to do what they don't want to do!" another end of that declaration is," the greater the hypnosis, the more they need to do it! The more you want to quit, the greater the success and, obviously, the less motivation, the less success you can expect! "Your readiness to understand instructions is the next concern. To be mesmerized, you have to put aside everything you've ever heard about hypnosis. And if you've been mesmerized without performance previously, the anticipated progress has almost little to do with it. Hypnosis has too many factors facilitating performance or dis-allowing progress. Hypnotherapy is strongly contextual. All may describe this differently. Every hypnotherapist must pick their own tool. Nobody is correct or incorrect, but like paintings, they can choose what they want. They may well be the country's best hypnotherapist, and a buddy has advised you to go there. If you're not happy with their style or appearance, though, you may not do the same as your mate. So remain optimistic and consider another hypnotherapist who can meet your hopes. So many times, I said, "I've tried hypnotherapy, and it really doesn't fit for me!" I believe everyone should aspire to be good through hypnosis, and they can aspire to play an instrument.

Next, you have to have a good attitude. This implies removing any reasoning or critique from your head, which will keep up your progress. People who use hypnotherapy also try to overanalyze or condemn what they don't think about. "I don't think I can be mesmerized, or I don't think this will work for me!" How can you deny or critique something you don't know about at all. In closing, get ready to be a non-smoker. Imagine what not craving a cigarette would have been like. Learn to feel what's going around a smoke inside your head. I assume hypnotherapy would do the best if you're able to stop smoking. You just need to imagine of one objective. What is that goal you'd like to enjoy after being hypnotized that you don't need to smoke? That can seem like a ridiculous question at first. You know what that feels like to want a smoke. Think about what not to crave a cigarette would feel like. You'll be effective once you have the response.

Hypnosis achieves little but to suppress the desire for smoking. You'll need your urge to smoke out! Then for a number of weeks after you've been hypnotized, you'll need to do hypnosis each day. The more important you were to cigarettes, the longer you will have to practice self-hypnosis, or perhaps be hypnotized again. For achievement some addicts may demand up to three exercises. Self-hypnosis seems to be your pencil eraser. It's trying to erase the impulses and cigarette behaviors. The deeper this is imprinted, the further you ought to delete it.

From early morning to even before bed, you can do hypnosis at any time. I typically recommend that you start self-hypnosis before bed. Self-hypnosis is similar to practice. Many of us do not like the exercises, the routines, or the hours of work. We despair at the thought of needing to do it on a daily basis. This gets more pleasurable by having self-hypnosis at dusk; when you lie down to go to bed. Self-hypnosis calls for a calm moment. Lying down is typically necessary, and duration of time to reach a feeling of relaxation that exists in our conscious well before sleeping and keeping it for a few minutes. Every one of these encounters exists a little before sleep, with next to no troubles.

- Lie comfortably, and shut your eyes.

- Build a sensation inside your mind as though you have lost the urge to smoke. This is known as "Purpose." Target is the mystical force that seems to be saying, "You did it!" In our vocabulary, the term purpose is always used to mean that we did so. Intention to buy or intention to murder is legally valid promises that claim you have achieved so in your view.

- Establish purpose as you shut your eyes, and you don't smoke anymore. This is your mind's might. Feeling like it would!

- Take very deep, long breaths.

Breathing has long been a key component of your tobacco consumption. Have you ever been drinking without being inhaled? Every cigarette requires approximately ten drags on a person. If you smoke a cigarette a day, you inhale about 200 times a day. Any pattern that you repeat 200 times a day is going to have huge strength.

- Through starting your self-hypnosis with a couple of slow breaths, you'll feel the relief cigarettes might have offered you in the old world for a fresh non-smoking relationship. It would be a chance to build your own key or mental memory to remove the need for smoking.

- Re-writing the hard-drive is the first move. Slowly start calming your body from the foot to your shoulders, after having a few deeper breaths. You can feel more relaxed up to your foot from your back. Any method should put you into the same feeling you had before you mesmerized yourself. That is why it is considered self-hypnosis. You are giving

yourself hypnosis. This is a ton like the daily playing of the instrument.

Without the exercise, you'll quickly forget the hypnosis experience, as you'd forget the soundtrack learning experience. You'll most certainly actually sleep until you're done. It is nice to sleep after hypnosis. Experts have a clear explanation of why going to sleep is great for smoking cessation hypnosis.

The feeling you have on falling asleep can impact your dreams. The visions influence the way you behave when you wake up, and your day would be influenced by the feeling you have when you wake up. In the past, you might have noticed if you fall asleep upset about something which is hard to relax and fall asleep. You most definitely got exhausted when you wake up in the morning. Most definitely, the day after was stressful. Then imagine falling asleep from the idea of smoking with your mind removed. Without any of the thought of smoke, you will wake up refreshed.

Steps of Self-Hypnosis for quitting smoking

1. Start by recognizing undesirable behavior. (It's Smoking in this case.)

2. Take the time to spot which indications or triggers will prompt you into those behavioral patterns.

- Is it that you have a smoke with your drink just after dinner?

- Do you often have a smoke when you get back to the house or if you take a break for lunch?

- Perhaps you light up anytime you meet friends?

- Maybe, is your nicotine addiction a reaction to pressure?

- But whatever signs you've got, you need to recognize them. Write them down.

3. Then you can use the strength of mind and intuition to envision yourself and change your reaction to certain indications. Just envision a situation in which this natural practice happens-such as walking out during the coffee break to smoke cigarettes. Now, start replacing that with a good picture, one that involves a payoff such as being unconcerned regarding your exhale or the stench of the smoking or how you'd use it more constructively for 15 minutes, and so on.

4. Re-iterating this visual picture starts to assist and guide the mind toward this daily behavior while in a calm position. The behavior management strategy of Neuro-linguistic training

will also improve this behavior change phase.

5. In combination with those methods, you could also use the code phrase Positive transformation hypnotherapy method.

5.6 Affirmations

I am taking my life into my hands.

I'm taller than cigarettes.

I am not a cigarette abuser.

I am very motivated to quit smoking.

My goal here is to be well.

I just don't like smoking.

I respect my body and care for it.

My lungs are tobacco-free.

I stopped smoking effectively.

My lungs are powerful and vibrant.

I take a free and deep breath.

I enjoy running (cycling, biking, hiking and so on. Use some aerobics).

I will break up old habits.

I'm introducing new good practices every day, in every way.

Every day, I am becoming stronger and better in every way.

Now I lead a smoke-free life.

I love to live a smoke-free life.

My natural condition is that of a no-smoker

My body feels safe and tidy as I stick to my good behaviors.

People respect my power of commitment and endorse my desire to lead a smoke-free existence.

My senses are strong, and I like to taste and smell the food to the maximum.

Smoking really doesn't appeal to me.

Each day my health gets better.

My lungs are packed with oxygen, and my muscles function well.

Eating in a non-smoking setting is excellent.

Chapter 6: Hypnosis Tips And Tricks And Weight Loss

The fundamentals of self-hypnosis are technically easy but still hard in reality. There are many helpful tips that you can employ n order to reap the full benefits of a hypnosis session, whether it's self-hypnosis or a guided one. Following are the tips:

Here are a few suggestions and strategies for self-hypnosis which you may try:

1. Use an Audiotape

If you're having a difficult time entrancing yourself, then use audio hypnosis of yourself to get you into the state of trance. There are lots of various forms of hypnosis audio tapes you can listen to at fair rates for free on the internet or pay for. Many self-hypnosis audios are essentially advertised as "hypnosis" audios. "Which are literally that the recording is captured by a skilled hypnotist so you will listen to it anytime you'd like? Since you are all by yourself in self-hypnosis and not working with a hypnotherapist, it's considered self-hypnosis. Audios by professional hypnotists like Dick

Sutphen or Rick Collingwood can be heard for a number of subjects, from becoming older to fighting over pollen allergies or asthma.

2. Create Your Own Audio Hypnosis

If you cannot find audio hypnosis with the specific recommendations you'd like, you can start making yourself. Online hypnosis texts may also be identified and you can change for your own needs. Document yourself (or have a buddy record it for you) and use it for audio hypnosis of yourself. Ensure that your recommendations are pleasant and in the current tense. You may use the "You're getting stronger and better" instruction form or an "I'm getting progressively better" reinforcement type.

3. Focus on Your Breathing

Take a yoga tip: Concentrate on your breath. Use long, deep, slow inhalations and even shorter exhales. Count your breath and exhale. This can help calm your mind down and effectively and efficiently bring you into a trance-like state.

4. Write Your Suggestions

Before you initiate your practice, get focused on what your entrancing recommendations would be. Keep them right beside you. If you decide to take a look at the hypnotic tips

during the self-hypnosis session and then replay them in your head while you shut your eyes again.

5. Memorize the Suggestions in Mind

The next move is to memorize the hypnotic ideas – so that would also integrate those recommendations into the sub-consciousness ever further.

6. Do a Slow and Easy Yoga Exercise

Originally the whole intent of yoga vipassana was to settle down the body so that it could sit for long periods of mindfulness. You will be very well fully ready for self-hypnosis and mindfulness by yoga practice-the the slow and controlled kind, not the heavily hyped European exercise yoga.

7. Listen to Binaural Beats When Hypnotizing Yourself

Binaural beats audios are audios built for the purposes of therapy and trance to carry the brain waves down into another zone. You're going to want to use binaural beats to take the brain into the wave state of theta. Many are, and are, on YouTube. For the best effect, use the headphones.

8. Try Self EMDR (Desensitization and Reprocessing in Eye Movement)

EMDR (Eye muscle movement Desensitization and Reprocessing) is a neurological procedure involving turning the head to the right and left when experiencing a question or trauma. You may execute EMDR on your own using video or audio, which moves from one part of the brain to another. Or you can only switch your eyes through self-hypnosis from side to side and see what happens.

9. Include EFT Prior To Your Self-Hypnosis Session

EFT is the short form of "Emotional Freedom Techniques," and it's an easy-to-learn acupressure form that involves pressing on junction (energy) places while concentrating on a problem. Adding EFT at the beginning of your hypnosis task will make it a lot easier to get into the daze and enhance its efficacy.

10. Add a Mantra to Use

Not clear what to do in the hypnotic state with yourself? Utilize a catchphrase. You may pick a typical phrase to use, such as Omm Mane Padme Hum, or start coming up with a whole phrase in English (or your mother tongue), such as "I am calm and happy." Return to it if your mind drifts through self-hypnosis.

11. Practice and Exercise daily

The best overall way to get ahead at self-hypnosis is by doing it every day. You can also do it in small bursts a few minutes a day. Consistently keep it at maximum performance. You will also note that it can be difficult to learn first, but when you move along, you get stronger. Maybe you'll start with guided audio hypnosis, but you'll soon be able to go off alone. Keep running!

12. Use Hypnotic Visual Imaging

This is how the technique works:

- Sit in a relaxed position with uncrossed feet and legs.

- Select a spot on the roof without rotating your neck or compressing your neck and focus your eyes on that stage. While keeping your eyes adjusted on that point, take some deep breaths, and keep it for as long as comfortable as possible. Then, as you exhale, repeat the statement, "My eyes are tired and heavy, and I want to SLEEP NOW." Repeat this process to yourself a few more times and, if your eyes had not already done so, let them shut and loosen up in a normal, closed place.

- Just like a rag doll, let your body become loose and relaxed in the chair. Then, slowly and intentionally, silently count down from five to nil. Tell yourself you're getting more and more confident with each and every list.

- Picture a picture that reflects a condition that you want to conquer and imagine yourself attaining your goal.

- Repeat an optimistic suggestion to yourself three to four times, like:

"I'm feeling optimistic, peaceful, and comfortable."

State it with confidence as you imagine the picture for 30 seconds or so.

Reiterate this three to four times and stay in hypnosis between times, and focus on relaxing your body.

- Return to space by counting one to five, then raising your eyes.

6.1 Law Of Attraction Affirmations

Attraction law authorities advocate utilizing constructive affirmations nearly unanimously. You may have been struggling to develop affirmations that function for you, though. Alternatively, maybe you're new to the Rule of Attraction and aren't sure how to continue finding the most effective method to train your subconscious mind to use constructive everyday affirmations. And though you might realize they are meant to be an effective device, perhaps you just don't grasp how statements function best and are afraid you're restricting the capacity for realization. Simply put, the explanation of affirmations uses 'positive sentences you revise to yourself' to build the subconscious mind's self-belief. This means making a catalog of statements effectively that encourage and inspire people to be good, improve, and overcome internal barriers as well as self-doubt. Here's how to use positive statements:

- Take gentle long deep breaths while inhaling and exhaling to 10.

- Stand before a mirror, and look in the eyes. If it comes easy, Smile.

- Talk the acknowledgment gradually and simply (or collection of meaningful statements).

- Repeat the statement(s) 3-5 times, truly concentrating on the significance of each word.

Affirmations for Health, Wealth and Happiness

I am thankful to just have experienced this very day when I reflect back today.

My failure becomes a moment to reflect.

My obstacles are Growth Paths.

Pleasure and tranquility take charge.

I and seeing how far I have already come, and I am able to move beyond my ambitions or desires.

I let go of the frivolous feelings or focus on the mistakes.

I am letting go of any apprehension or distress, and I accept a sense of peace.

I believe everything in my life would be a divine command.

I am thankful for all that I have in me, and for the ability to make the most of it.

I feel so fantastic, and for the rest of the day, I will enjoy that feeling.

"I am embracing my strength."

"These are plentiful and filling aspects of my existence."

"Any knowledge and I have is great for growth."

"I deserve to be respected. All around me is love.'

6.2 Multi-Sensory Programming Hypnosis

Hypnosis is also related to utilizing language and use relevant terms correctly. However, in actuality, as research shows, only the tiniest speck of our communication goes via words, while the greater part goes through non-verbal elements. We may use our shared nonverbal contact codes and components to put people further into a trance than any state they've ever felt. Each term that we use in our everyday speech has a non-verbal sense and the terms remain only as metaphors for items or other non-verbal codes.

Through a multi-sensory hypnotic induction, the nonverbal dialog should be implemented for three main reasons:

- Considering the emotional engagement of clients

- Bring it to adjust its operating scheme

- Offer non-verbal suggestions

For convenience's sake, we will divide the various non - verbal components we may use into sections:

Paralinguistic — Pitch, tone of voice and possessing the influence of meaningless expressions

Proxemics — the use of space and motion to create a social bond

Kinesic and Gaze — Hand movements; the hypnotic passes; the gaze's social meaning

Digital - Explore the special power of contact

Each conversational induction typically uses some of the above-mentioned elements, but perhaps the most crucial thing is to incorporate them all together in such a powerful and influential combination at the same time as awareness, which is the most helpful at a given moment. The "rapport" we can get using elements is so good that any behavioral improvement actually occurs more effectively and rapidly than through some other process.

The reason for this powerful "relationship" is because we don't interact on the exterior (as if we just use words); conversely, we interact on a deeper and deeper level that includes the client emotionally. Via hypnotherapy, you will help restore reflexes to keep you gratified and bring that wonderful sense of well-being into play.

6.3 Hypnotic Gastric Band For Weight Loss

The hypnotic gastric band process works by employing visualization techniques when in a trance-like state. Some may ask how strong a simulation they are. It is very easy, indeed. Try out that experiment. Only ask at your front entrance. Which side's on the lock? You called an image of your purchase to mind to answer that question.

It is mental imagery, and all of us can do it. Visualization will influence the body dramatically. When you visualize a painful situation, your body produces cortisol and your skeletal system contracts. Whenever you think about a relaxing thing, the chemicals in our bodies will change, and the muscular system calms down.

Similarly, anytime you think you've had a surgery where the stomach has narrowed from an equivalent of a cantaloupe to equivalent of a golf ball; it literally affects the body's signaling system, so that you start to feel completely satisfied after just a few mouthfuls. Even though it sounds ridiculous because you are aware of what's happening, the mind-body connection behaves as if you had it, and there's an actual latex ring on your stomach.

A collection of hormones regulates digestion, and several perform multiple tasks. For e.g., GLP1, which informs your brain you've had plenty to eat, often delays secretion of the stomach acid. The main thing is that it not only reduces your stomach size but also carefully recalibrates the leptin inducing processes that are responsible for your satiety.

That's why it's so efficient, as it plays a hand-on role with such interconnected processes that our brains control. On a physiological level, the internal gastric band can recalibrate the sense of fullness.

- Firstly, recall an instance where you felt completely loaded to the point of being uneasy, and perhaps you felt sluggish and even felt like vomiting.

- Recall another time a day; you felt very hungry to the point that you felt like starving in your stomach. Your stomach seemed hollow and growling with hunger.

During the Hypnotic Gastric Band self-hypnosis audio, the subconscious accesses these memories to reconfigure the sense of fullness and make you aware of the phases that lie in the middle of hunger and stuffiness. As a consequence of the Hypnotic Gastric Unit, the unconscious mind will make the fullness flow swifter, louder and more urgent.

Conclusion

In this book, we looked in detail at the very many benefits of deep sleep hypnosis and how it can be used to treat a plethora of problems. To sum it up, we started off with an in-depth analysis of deep sleep hypnosis. We talked extensively about the basics of hypnosis, what it is, and how it's done. We now know the different stages of hypnosis, i.e., induction, hypnotic, and post-hypnotic suggestions. Then, we described and debunked a few myths related to hypnosis. Afterward, there was a subtopic dedicated to the power of our subconscious mind and how we can use auto-suggestion to re-frame it. Then, the chapter went deep into the benefits of hypnosis for insomnia, smoking, and medical illnesses.

The second chapter was all about hypnosis as the cure for overthinking. We introduced the three types of overthinking, which include regret, future worry, and analysis paralysis. We also mentioned a list of daily affirmations to fight back overthinking and anxiety, along with a sleep hypnosis script for you to follow along. The chapter closed with some valuable mindfulness tips. In the next chapter, we also learned a lot about how low self-esteem is developed in the first place and what is the power of our self-loathing repetitive words along with tips on developing positive self-talk. We also included a self-hypnosis script for you to follow before going to sleep. Finally, the chapter closed with helpful daily affirmations to build confidence.

Moreover, we discussed all past lives and the tell-tale signs of you having a past life. These included weird birthmarks, certain passions, unexplained pain, and bizarre dreams, etc. then we looked at the efficacy of Past Life Regression Therapy (PLRT) to heal traumas, access past lives, and recover their memories. We then moved on to smoking cessation, the power of our subconscious mind, and why willpower only goes so far in addiction recovery. We also learned a few mindfulness techniques for quitting smoking, along with a hypnosis script and a list of daily affirmations. In the final chapter, we closed the book with a list of some tips and tricks everyone doing self-hypnosis should use. We also looked at the latest trend in hypnosis for weight loss, i.e., the hypnotic gastric band. We included a long list of daily affirmations for health, wealth, and happiness, which use the power of the law of attraction. Finally, we ended the book with how Multi-Sensory Programming Hypnosis works through non-verbal communication rather than the spoken words used in typical hypnosis.

Glossary

Hypnosis: Also named the hypnotic condition that is a comfortable, intensely concentrated frame of mind you enter after becoming hypnotized.

Hypnotism: The mechanism by which the hypnotic condition was triggered. A traditional entrancing stimulation may require intense relaxation, eye closing, and counting.

Hypnotherapy: Hypnotherapy relates to the usage of treatment with hypnosis and hypnotism. Hypnotists are qualified practitioners who utilize hypnosis to support people to achieve improvement targets.

Suggestion: It's a hypnotic or subconscious integration of an idea initiated by one.

Insomnia: Persistent sleeplessness

Overthinking: It's a condition when someone thinks too much or too long about a particular thing.

Analysis Paralysis: Analysis Paralysis (or paralysis due to analysis) explains a person or group process when over-analysis or overthinking of a scenario can lead to a "paralysis" of the forward movement or decision-making," which means that no remedy or plan of action is decided.

Subconscious: It is in or around the portion of the mind about which one is not entirely aware but which affects one's behavior and feelings.

Mindfulness: A mental condition attained by concentrating one's mind on the current moment while peacefully acknowledging and embracing one's emotions, perceptions, and physical stimuli, employed as a therapeutic tool.

Self-talk: An internal voice, also called self-talk, inner expression, inner debate, or inner debate, is the inner voice of an individual who, though awake, provides a running verbal monolog of thoughts.

Self-hypnosis: Self-hypnosis or auto-hypnosis is a shape, a mechanism, or the product of a hypnotic self-induced condition.

Regression: It is a shift to a previous state or a less developed one.

Past Life Regression Therapy (PLRT): Restoration of past existence is a method that utilizes hypnosis to recreate what therapists consider to be images of previous lives or incarnations.

Trauma: A deeply distressing experience.

Addiction: The fact or condition that a particular substance or activity is addicted to.

Willpower: Control to do something, or to restrict impulses.

Gastric Band: In the clinical management of obesity, a latex device is installed around the upper part of the stomach generating a small pouch just above the latex band and thus limiting the quantity of food that can be comfortably consumed.

References

1. How Hypnosis Works. Retrieved from **https://science.howstuffworks.com/science-vs-myth/extrasensory-perceptions/hypnosis2.htm**

2. 5 Powerful Auto Suggestion Techniques To Take Control Of Your life. Retrieved from **https://www.mindtosucceed.com/auto-suggestion-techniques.html**

3. **How to Stop Analysis Paralysis.** Retrieved from **https://www.hypnosisdownloads.com/thinking-skills/analysis-paralysis**

4. What Is Cellular Memory? 8 Signs Of A 'Past Life' Connection. Retrieved from **https://www.thelawofattraction.com/cellular-memory-past-life/**

5. Self-talk and negative 'hypnosis'. Retrieved from **https://nlp-now.co.uk/self-talk-negative-hypnosis/**

6. Hypnosis For Memory Retrieval. Retrieved from **https://www.hypnotherapyandmeditation.com/services/hypnosis-for-memory-retrieval/**

7. The Psychology Behind Chronic Overthinking (and How to Stop It). Retrieved from **https://www.mydomaine.com/overthinking-hacks**

8. How Can You Get a Sounder Sleep With Hypnotherapy? Retrieved from **https://www.verywellhealth.com/hypnosis-for-sleep-disorders-89676**